Life Support

Diary of an ICU Doctor on the Frontline of the Covid Crisis

JIM DOWN

PENGUIN BOOKS

PENGUIN BOOKS

UK | USA | Canada | Ireland | Australia
India | New Zealand | South Africa

Penguin Books is part of the Penguin Random House group of companies
whose addresses can be found at global.penguinrandomhouse.com.

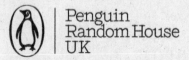

Penguin
Random House
UK

First published by Viking 2021
Published with a new afterword in Penguin Books 2021
001

Typeset by Jouve (UK), Milton Keynes
Printed and bound in Great Britain by Clays Ltd, Elcograf S.p.A.

The authorized representative in the EEA is Penguin Random House Ireland,
Morrison Chambers, 32 Nassau Street, Dublin D02 YH68

A CIP catalogue record for this book is available from the British Library

ISBN: 978-0-241-50632-5

www.greenpenguin.co.uk

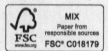

Life

'An extraordinarily frank book laced with humour
and self-deprecation' *The Times*

'Down is an ideal narrator . . . Three quarters of the way through
Life Support I started weeping' Tanya Gold, *Daily Telegraph*

'Deeply affecting – a personal memoir that grips, harrows, inspires and,
ultimately, uplifts with its vein of deep humanity' Philippe Sands

'One of the doctors with the most hands-on experience of Covid
in the country' Edward Docx, *New Statesman*

'A deeply moving and beautifully written account of what life was truly
like for our frontline ICU teams during the first wave of COVID-19'
Dr Kevin Fong

'Reading *Life Support* I was gripped, amazed, appalled and, ultimately,
inspired. If Jim Down is as good a doctor as he is a writer,
I'd definitely want him treating me' John O'Farrell

'I can't think of a more important and compulsive book to come
out of the "Plague Year". Read and weep with gratitude for the
NHS and doctors like Jim Down' Rachel Johnson

'Jim Down's *Life Support* is essential reading for everyone who has been
affected by COVID-19, which is to say everyone. Beautifully written, it
combines warmth, humour and science to give a portrait of one of the
most important but least understood parts of any hospital by one of
the UK's pre-eminent ICU physicians' Dr Chris van Tulleken

'Reading this, I felt humbled. Written with great clarity, as well as
humour and compassion, this is an extraordinary account of life on the
Covid frontline, of the expertise and the dogged, unending labour of
those who attempt to keep the rest of us – however sceptical we are,
however careless – alive' Lissa Evans, author of *V for Victory*

'This is the struggle against COVID-19 unfolding in real time . . . It is a story of how some of our most gifted and dedicated medical practitioners have been brought to the very edge of their abilities and endurance and how they came through, scarred but wiser . . . Above all it is a very human story about how people – medics and patients alike – found common cause in the face of a nasty speck of a disease that threatens our way of life' George Alagiah

'An honest and engaging eyewitness account of the Covid crisis from one of London's busiest intensive care units, that demonstrates the compassion and dedication of frontline staff dealing with a terrible new disease. It should be required reading for anyone who wants to understand why our lives have been turned upside down by the pandemic' Fergus Walsh, Medical Editor, BBC

'*Life Support* immediately transported me back to those early days of uncertainty, the growing fear as the waves lapped our feet, and then the frantic struggle to stay above water as the tsunami broke. The reader will learn a deal more about intensive care units and the jobs of the people who work there. But this book is far from a technical manual. It is a human narrative – and an important one' Hugh Montgomery, Professor of Intensive Care Medicine, UCL, and author of *Control*

'Brought me to tears' *Financial Times*

ABOUT THE AUTHOR

Dr Jim Down is a consultant in critical care and anaesthesia at University College London Hospitals. He chairs the ICU consultants' group, the department of anaesthesia weekly scientific meetings and the UCLH Trust guideline committee. During the COVID-19 pandemic he has been on a new full-time, full-shift clinical rota for ICU, and was appointed Trust Lead for Ethics. This is his first book.

To Mum and Dad

Contents

24 March 2020

'Jim, they need you in bay 5. The young guy – Adam – in bed 36 has crashed his blood pressure.'

'Right, OK. Thanks.' I walked back to the table of personal protective equipment (PPE), dropped my valuables into the tray and picked a new mask from the box.

'Has his temp gone up again?'

'Don't know. I'll ask.' Taciana, the staff nurse who'd called me, spoke into her walkie-talkie.

'Jim's coming in. What's his temperature? In bed 36.'

The walkie-talkie crackled.

'What?' she asked again. 'Sorry, can you repeat that?'

'41.8.'

'Shit,' I muttered, adjusting the mask under my chin. I felt sick. I'd seen Adam that morning on the ward round and set up a plan, so why was he so hot again? He was a young man, still in his twenties; his whole life was ahead of him. This was meant to be a disease of the old and frail. His next of kin was his mum. She was probably my age, but I'd not met her. Relatives weren't allowed in during Covid. He had a six-year-old son too, called Harry. This was not supposed to be happening. His temperature should have settled with the measures we'd put in place. Viruses make you hot, but not this hot. This was like a drug reaction to ecstasy or one of the anaesthetic gases: malignant hyperthermia. He was life-threateningly hot again, and now his blood pressure was crashing.

I took three breaths in and out to check the mask's seal. Air blew into my eyes, so I adjusted the strap and squeezed the metal band tight around the bridge of my nose.

What next?

I glanced at the laminated PPE donning guide – hat.

As I pushed my arms into the waterproof gown, I tried to think logically. Cool him first then go from there. I pulled a second pair of gloves over the first and taped them to the gown.

'Taciana, can you tell them to cool him with whatever they've got – wet towels, bladder irrigation, ice packs, fluids. And if there's another consultant around, can you ask them to join me?'

Next came the plastic apron and finally a grey visor from the tray. The black ones gave me a headache within twenty minutes.

My consultant colleague Rik joined me at the donning table and began the laborious process. It was three tables in fact, hastily set up in a row like trestle cake stands at a village fête. They took up most of the corridor outside the ICU bays, each piled high with boxes of masks, aprons, hats, gloves and visors. Underneath were more boxes, and downstairs hundreds more. Short strips of tape created a fringe around the edge of each table, pre-prepared to stick gloves to gowns. At the far end a large plastic tray overflowed with sandwich bags filled with the valuables of staff currently 'donned' within the Covid bays.

I patted my chest, mentally checking off the items of PPE.

'I'll tie you up.'

Someone I'd never seen before tied the back of my gown and apron.

'Thanks.' I mumbled, then raised my voice. 'Can we get the Doppler and Echo machine into bay 5? And the crash trolley. And . . . can you keep someone at the door for communication?'

I checked the tapes on my gloves one final time.

'And can you call his mother?' I shouted to no one in particular. 'And say?'

'Come in.'

1. Beginning

January – March 2020

I had always assumed I would become a GP. I saw myself as a people person and I had visions of living in a village by the sea with a wife, kids and a dog, working in a small friendly GP practice. I'd have Wednesday afternoons off, watch my kids play sport and in the summer take them dinghy sailing down an estuary, to a pub perhaps. If not a pillar of the local community, I'd certainly be an active member of it. It was usually summer in my imagined future, but the short spells of winter were spent on crisp, cold walks along the beach under a low sun.

And then I did my medical student GP placement and realized that I didn't have the nerve or the patience. I couldn't cope with the lack of certainty, the inability to get to the bottom of every problem and the necessity for calculated risks. The fact that you had to send people away knowing that one in a thousand might have cancer was too much for me. I wanted to scan them all from head to foot. It also became apparent that I wasn't quite the 'people person' I'd thought I was. I left the placement with a new level of respect for GPs and a gaping hole of a career plan.

ICU and anaesthesia only really crossed my mind as possibilities when I was a surgical house doctor in Exeter. Less than a year qualified, I was living by the sea, even sailing occasionally, and ever surer that a surgical career was not for me, but the anaesthetists and intensivists intrigued me. They were confident, cheerful and unflappable. They understood physiology and pharmacology in a way other doctors had long forgotten and seemed to approach medicine from first principles rather than by pattern recognition and a dropdown list of possible diagnoses. They could manipulate that physiology in front of your eyes and most impressively they swept up my sickest patients and magically cured them on the ICU. They also seemed to enjoy life. They talked about things outside of medicine and spent what I deemed a healthy amount of time in the sea or on Dartmoor.

Many people choose pure anaesthesia (or pure ICU), but a proportion do both, and the combination appealed to me. The chaos and excitement of ICU would be offset by time in the operating theatre, undisturbed and focused on a single patient. Within a year I was back in Exeter to start my training. Two years later I had finished the first stage of my training, I was single (surrounded by smug marrieds), and my watersports career seemed to consist mainly of breaking other people's equipment, so with nothing to lose I decided to give London a go. After six tough months in a West London ICU, I got offered higher (registrar) training in North Central London. University College Hospital (UCH) was at the heart of the rotation. I loved the place and I never looked back.

My first ICU consultant meeting at UCH was on 7 July 2005. We sat down in the brand-new ICU seminar room in the brand-new hospital at 9 a.m., but by 9.20 I was back on my Vespa, scooting across town to the Royal London (where I was still officially working) to help deal with casualties of the London bombings. We admitted nine victims to the Royal London ICU that day, eight of whom survived, but many lost limbs and suffered life-changing, long-term injuries. I left that job a few weeks later, thinking and hoping that I'd never see anything so devastating again.

Five years later I gave evidence at the Independent Inquest of the bombings and met the parents of the patient who'd died on our unit. At the end of the day they hugged me and thanked me for setting their minds at rest. Ever since the day he'd died, they'd worried that more could have been done for their son and that they should have fought harder. Now they were convinced that we'd done everything possible and were optimistic they would be able find some sort of peace. It had taken five years, but finally they had closure. I was relieved for them but also left wondering how many other relatives carry around that doubt and guilt for years after the death of a loved one on ICU.

I enjoyed the Royal London ICU. It was chaotic and exciting, because you never knew when the helicopter might land and what poor injured soul it would deliver, but it was also exhausting. By the end of my year there I had begun to dread the *thud thud thud* of the approaching chopper and, although I missed it when I left, I was pleased to settle into the relative order and calm of life at UCH, where stabbings and traffic accidents were replaced by designer drug overdoses, oncology and tropical diseases. I've been there ever since.

I first encountered COVID-19 in January 2020. Our Intensive Care Unit is split over two sites, the main thirty-five-bedded unit at UCH and a nine-bedded satellite unit in Westmoreland Street Hospital in Marylebone. At any one time two intensive care consultants cover the UCH unit and a third is dispatched to Westmoreland Street to care for patients following their major thoracic and urological surgery. I enjoy my weeks at Westmoreland Street. It has its moments, but it's a small, elective hospital, so the pace is generally slower, and the Marylebone location means access to some excellent coffee shops.

On 3 January 2020 I was sitting in the Westmoreland Street ICU office, contemplating some after-work sales shopping, when Professor Sir Alimuddin Zumla popped in to do his round. Rubbing shoulders with world leaders in their field is a perk of working at UCH. Two of my close colleagues have been on *Desert Island Discs* (terrible song choices), a third is one of the doctors to the royal family, and Chris Whitty passed through ICU on his ward round just a week or two before taking up his new role as chief medical officer (I'd had no idea). I applied to work at UCH because it was filled with people I both liked and respected, but the fact that I bump into professors, medical policy advisors, journal editors and general movers and shakers at every turn is an unexpected bonus.

Quietly spoken and unassuming, Ali Zumla is an international expert in infectious and tropical diseases, but part of his day job is to advise on infection in the Westmoreland Street ICU. We talked through the patients, changed some antibiotics, wished each other a happy new year and were about to part company when he said, 'There's a coronavirus outbreak in China, you know.'

'Uh huh,' I replied, my mind back on the bargains I might pick up in Selfridges.

'Wuhan city. Nasty.'

'Right.'

Looking back, I am slightly ashamed that I didn't take more interest in the conversation. It was clearly bothering him, but we'd had several coronavirus scares over the years (SARS, MERS, etc.), and they'd all come to nothing as far as the UK was concerned. I remember losing sleep over SARS, and when I did sleep dreaming of a post-apocalyptic world in which we walked the streets in Hazmat suits. I had no desire to revisit those nightmares. Wuhan was a long way away, and I had shirts to buy.

Through most of January my relationship with the virus was very much like everyone else's. I swung between 'Oh my God, this is unimaginable,' and 'Nah, it'll probably never happen.'

Then, in the last week of the month, I was away at a medical conference. The Covid news items were becoming more frequent, and it had crept into the dinner-table conversation, although still way behind Brexit, gossip and climate change in the pecking order. There was one delegate, however, who was taking it very seriously. I don't know if he'd studied it in more depth or was just naturally pessimistic, but he was in no doubt; this was coming and it was going to be devastating.

But life carried on as usual. We took the children to France for the February half term to visit my sister and her family and if we did talk about Covid it was only in abstract terms. We were much more concerned about our childrens' screen time and our mother's health. We moaned about Boris Johnson's Brexit plans and worried how they might affect my sister's future in France, but it never crossed our minds that Covid might separate us for the next six months. We made a firm arrangement to meet up again for the summer half term.

In the first week of March, however, the ICUs in northern Italy started to fill up with Covid patients, and, despite the UK still being in the 'containment' phase of its response, the virus had reached all four corners of the country. On 2 March the UK reported its first Covid death, and while some colleagues were still referring to it as 'just a nasty flu outbreak', many of us were starting to get nervous. Once into a community, this virus seemed to spread fast, and it clearly made many people extremely sick.

My personal position shifted significantly when I paused to think seriously about the mortality rate. There was a lot of conflicting information at the time, but the death rate most commonly quoted in the media and around the hospital was 3 per cent. That was thirty times the mortality of seasonal flu, which already put a huge strain on our ICU bed capacity. How on earth would we cope with something potentially as widespread and thirty times as deadly?

And what about the risk to our own health? Doctors tend to split into stoics and hypochondriacs. I think it's the nature of the job. Seeing so much disease pushes you one way or the other, and sadly I am in the hypochondriac camp. I have developed some techniques to manage this (mainly running around Hampstead Heath at all hours of the day and night), but the only times I felt truly safe at medical school were during my gynaecology and paediatric placements – at last some illnesses that I definitely didn't have. My default position is that I will probably not only catch, but also be killed by, most potentially fatal diseases, and Covid was no exception. I was male, heading for my fiftieth birthday and pre-diabetic (possibly). It did not look good.

On 3 March the Royal Free Hospital, a teaching hospital less than 2 miles from us, admitted its first Covid patient to ICU. There was no more denying it: the pandemic was coming, and it was time to prepare. We needed to work out not just how we'd cope with the arrival of patients, but also how we'd protect the staff. The Royal Free is a High Consequence Infectious Disease hospital and so had been designated a first receiving hospital for Covid. They already had experience with diseases that present a serious risk to staff, particularly the Ebola virus, so our clinical director, David Howell, telephoned Dan Martin, a Royal Free ICU consultant, and invited him to come and educate us the following Monday.

That weekend I travelled to Dorset to visit my parents. A handful of people with underlying health conditions had by now died of Covid, and reported cases were up to nearly 200, particularly concentrated around London, so I telephoned ahead to ask if they'd rather I didn't come. My father, also a doctor and a definite stoic, said absolutely not. He wasn't the slightest bit worried about the virus. My parents were physically fit, but at eighty-one and seventy-nine they were in a high-risk group, and my mother has rapidly progressing dementia.

On the Sunday of that weekend Mum and I went for a long walk in the hills around where they live, and as we began our final descent towards home she suddenly suggested we run.

'Run?'

'Shall we?' she asked, with a mix of confusion and excitement.

'Yeah, let's run.' I agreed, and so we did. We ran and leaped through the mud and the cowpats for hundreds of yards, like ten-year-olds. A huge grin spread across my mother's face.

On Monday I was on for the main ICU. Two of us cover the thirty-five ICU beds for a week at a time, in my case one week every month. I anaesthetize for operations and deliver my non-clinical activities during the other weeks, but the ICU weeks are my busiest. The seven days on starts with a telephone handover from the outgoing consultant on Sunday, which always reminds me of Sunday evenings as a child, when the fun stopped and I faced the reality of return to school. The run of seven consecutive days is intentional, to give us the chance to get to know the patients and their relatives properly so that we can make meaningful, shared decisions about ongoing plans, but it is tiring and unpredictable. We are on call every other night through that week and not infrequently called in at 3 a.m. to deal with emergencies. It is a daunting prospect each time, particularly the first couple of days, when we're still getting to know all the patients, but by day three I am usually into the swing of it and by the weekend, if I've slept, enjoying it. That week, however, I couldn't complain. I was only covering for a colleague until the Tuesday morning.

I arrived just before 8 a.m. on the Monday for our morning team brief, when all the nurses and doctors for the day shift (roughly forty-five people) squeeze into the ICU coffee room to hear 'highlights' from an outgoing night shift representative.

The big news of that brief was that we had admitted our first possible Covid patient. He was doing well: alert, chatting, stable on just facemask oxygen and crucially not on my end of the unit. It was, however, a wake-up call, and I was pleased that Dan was coming later that day to tell us all we needed to know. Otherwise the team brief was very much like any other. It had been a busy night, with three other admissions, but there'd been good teamwork (they always say that) and no disasters. There were four hotspots (two my end), and it was all rounded off with an inspirational quote by Maya Angelou: 'They may forget your name, but they will never forget how you made them feel.'

There is always a message of the week, and that week it was a reminder that everyone must get FFP3 mask (a facemask with a viral filter) fit tested. A good seal around the FFP3 mask was deemed crucial for staff safety, and if the mask didn't fit you needed to shave off your beard (if you had one) or request a fully sealed hood instead. The hoods were not only terrifying to behold, they were also expensive and needed ordering.

I'd done my fit test the previous week but found it more confusing than I'd expected. The process started with a spray of scent to check that I could smell it without the mask, but I think I inhaled too deeply and was left with stinging nostrils and a lingering after-smell. I then donned my mask and over that a hood. My colleague Jane pumped twenty shots of scent into the hood and asked me whether I could smell them. If I could, the mask's fit was inadequate, but the problem was I couldn't tell. The after-smell from the test spray had never really gone away, so I wasn't sure if I was smelling new scent or old. We repeated the process with a different scent, but by now my nose was dry, and my smell centre completely baffled. I was starting to feel embarrassed and a bit nauseous, but the scent didn't seem to be getting stronger, and I needed to pick up the kids, so I said it was fine and was ticked off the list.

After a succinct handover from the night doctors, I dispatched them to their beds (they looked exhausted and would be back for another night shift in eleven hours) and set off on my morning ward round. I was on for the north half of the unit, which meant fewer beds (fifteen as opposed to twenty on south) but generally sicker, more complex patients.

ICU is the last truly general ward in the hospital because we admit patients from every specialty, but it doesn't look like a general ward. To the side of each bed are two large gantries, suspended from the ceiling. Piped oxygen, air and electric cables run through the gantries, and hanging off them are monitors, syringe drivers, a ventilator, suction and a computer terminal. There are often two or three other free-standing machines around the bed such as a 4-foot-high artificial kidney ('the filter'), a machine to monitor the output from the heart, a warming or cooling blanket and a chest of drawers on wheels stuffed with equipment. Even the beds themselves are impressive feats of engineering, with sophisticated air mattresses to reduce pressure sores and multiple settings to optimize patient care and comfort. It's a high-tech environment – but there are no TVs, and the wifi signal is awful. I don't know who designed the ICU, but they obviously felt that the half of our patients who are not sedated and ventilated could jolly well read a book or listen to the wireless.

If the function of one or more of a patient's vital organs (heart, lungs, kidneys, brain and liver) has deteriorated to the point that they require support or continuous monitoring and there is a reasonable chance of recovery, then we bring that patient into ICU. Broadly we, the intensivists, then look after the vital organs while their specialist 'home' team offer advice about the underlying disease.

Ten of the north beds of our ICU are single side rooms. They are used for a combination of vulnerable people who need protection from infections and those with the infections that we do not want to pass on to other patients (MRSA, Clostridium Difficile, etc.). One of the major specialties at UCH is haematology-oncology (blood cancer), and that Monday six of the ten side rooms contained patients with leukaemia or lymphoma who had recently received chemotherapy or a bone marrow transplant. These treatments are life-saving but also brutal and wreak havoc on the immune system, leaving the patients extremely vulnerable to a plethora of infections and complications. Four of those six were sedated on ventilators, and three were under forty years of age.

Of the other side rooms, one was empty, one was occupied by a man with severe pneumonia and infectious diarrhoea (ventilated via a tracheostomy but awake and impressively focused), another by a woman transferred from another hospital who'd vomited so much that she'd ruptured her gullet (four drains in place and awake with an ever-present fiancé) and the final one by an alcoholic in his fifties with liver failure and MRSA (ventilated and usually surrounded by three friends who smelled strongly of pub).

In my open bay I had a young woman who'd taken an overdose of her antidepressants (ventilated, but hopefully not for long), a man in his sixties with a stroke (breathing for himself, but drowsy with right-sided paralysis and impaired swallowing), a chronic bronchitic with superadded pneumonia (ventilated, but seemingly indestructible) and a forty-two-year-old who'd had an emergency colon resection for inflammatory bowel disease (reading the paper and ready for discharge to a normal ward). It was busy but manageable.

I spent the next three hours reviewing each of these patients in detail. I went over their stories again, examined each in turn, looked at their blood results, x-rays and scans, reviewed the sedation, blood pressure support and ventilator settings, checked the drug charts, talked to the specialists who'd referred them and set up plans for the next twenty-four hours.

Most of the patients were stable, but the woman in side room 5 was deteriorating fast. She was a lawyer in her fifties with a husband and three children in their early twenties. She had a nasty form of leukaemia that had relapsed following a bone marrow transplant and she was now on novel chemotherapy.

I'd met her with her older daughter (a family member was always at the bedside) two weeks previously, shortly after her admission to ICU. Back then she was still breathing for herself, albeit on high flow oxygen, but she was grey and puffy, and every breath looked like hard work.

'Good morning, Mrs Gooding, I'm Jim Down, one of the ICU consultants,' I'd ventured gently.

'Hello, Jim, lovely to meet you. It's Susan, please.' Her face lit up as she spoke, and her voice was crisp and precise.

'How are you?'

'Not too bad, all things considered.'

She turned to her daughter, squeezed her hand and smiled. Her daughter smiled back and wiped away a tear.

Susan had known from the start that she was in trouble. Her heart had been weakened by one of the chemotherapy agents, her white blood cells (required to fight infection) wiped out by another, and she'd seemed to go from one infection to the next. But despite all this, she'd remained engaged and positive, always keen to explore the next option. Ten days after I had seen her, however, she'd been hit by a particularly nasty bacteria and she'd deteriorated fast.

Now she was sedated and intubated with a tube that passed through her mouth down into her windpipe. A mechanical ventilator was delivering each breath via this tube, she was on the filter for her kidneys and requiring large doses of drugs to drive her heart and support her blood pressure. She was receiving the most powerful antibiotics we had, but still she continued to go downhill. She had no immune system to speak of, and her blood pressure was still falling. She looked awful: pale and sweaty and an angry rash covered her trunk. Added to all that, there were signs that she wasn't responding to the chemotherapy.

I fiddled with the ventilator, altered her blood pressure medication and arranged to meet with her family and the haematologist at 2.30 that afternoon. There was no way back for her now.

At 10.30 our microbiologist arrived, so I broke off the ward round again to sit down with him and go through the patients' infections and antibiotics.

There were also two minor emergencies (a partially blocked breathing tube and a sudden drop in blood pressure), but they were quickly resolved, and by 12.15 p.m. I had seen everyone (except the man with severe pneumonia, who'd been on the commode when I arrived, and the post-op patient who'd already escaped to the ward), so I ran to Pret a Manger and back in time for the 12.30 multi-disciplinary team (MDT) meeting in the seminar room.

The daily MDT is the chance for all groups (physiotherapists, pharmacists, dieticians, nurses and doctors) to say their piece. Each group individually plays a crucial role for the patients on ICU, and the chance for them to sit down and discuss things is vital. It should be focused and rapid fire and is scheduled to last forty-five minutes. Unfortunately, it is vulnerable to sabotage by professorial anecdote and can stretch well into the afternoon, but not on my weeks. At 1.14 p.m. precisely we wrapped up and welcomed Dan Martin and his nursing colleague from the Royal Free Hospital to tell us all they knew about Covid.

The ICU seminar room is small and seats twenty comfortably, twenty-five at a push, but that lunchtime there must have been forty of us crammed into the room and more spilling out into the corridor. It was the most popular meeting we'd held all year. Dan's primary brief was to demonstrate how to don and doff the personal protective equipment safely, but we planned to squeeze him for as much information as we could. He and his colleague beautifully demonstrated how to put on the layers of protection and then more importantly how to remove them without contaminating themselves. It was smooth, methodical and meticulous, but as soon as they'd finished we bombarded them with questions.

'Can you do it on your own?'

'What if you touch your face when doffing?'

'Can we keep valuables in our pockets?'

They suggested we have 'buddies' at the donning stations to check each stage of both processes, that we practise ahead of time and that valuables be left outside Covid areas. We should try not to touch our face, but if we did, we just needed to wash with soap and water.

Everything they said made sense and was almost exactly in line with our policy, except for one thing – shoes. The Royal Free used communal boots as part of their PPE. They had stocks on ICU and after each use the boots were decontaminated, but we were going to wear our own shoes. I wasn't happy about that. The process was all so careful and precise and yet we weren't going to change our shoes – why not? Did the virus not like smelly feet? I was informed that it was impractical to have so many communal boots (we'd never have the right sizes or be able clean them all) and that I should wipe down my shoes after each shift and keep a pair for hospital use only, but it all seemed a bit slapdash to me.

Over the next fifteen minutes I became obsessed with the shoe issue. People weren't giving me a satisfactory explanation, and I felt fobbed off. Months later I'm embarrassed, it seems ridiculous now, but it reflected my state of mind at the time. I was trying to rationalize the personal risk. As long as we were doing all we could to minimize the danger, then fine, let's get on with it, but this policy seemed illogical and foolhardy. If we were putting ourselves in harm's way then at the very least our protocols should be rigorous and watertight.

Dan also talked to us about the learning from the Royal Free Ebola experience. The threats to staff of Ebola and Covid were different: a few cases of an extremely deadly virus transmitted by direct contact, versus many cases of a less deadly virus transmitted via droplets and surfaces, but the lessons were nevertheless relevant. Staff safety must always be paramount, stethoscopes should not be used because of the risk of spreading the infection, and periods spent in PPE should be no longer than two hours, three at the absolute maximum. Dan has been to the top of Everest, he's made of stern stuff, but even he couldn't deal with the heat and discomfort of full PPE for more than three hours. Teams of staff would be needed outside 'dirty' Covid areas to replenish the PPE, fetch and carry, clean visors and help people to 'don' and 'doff' safely. Everything would be labour-intensive and time-consuming.

It was a sobering meeting. They suggested that we had a week before it hit us in earnest. Based on the expected number of hospital admissions, the estimation that 20 per cent of those would need ICU and a predicted five-day doubling rate we could expect to have a trickle of ICU cases that week, ten patients by the middle of the next week and twenty at the beginning of the week after. We listened, we nodded and we took notes, but still it was surreal. The week before we'd been arguing about the cost of new bins.

I walked out of the meeting behind my ICU consultant colleague, Rik.

'You all right?'

'Yeah.' Rik was miles away, deep in thought.

'Maybe it won't be as bad, as they think,' I said, trying to convince myself as much as him.

'Hmm.'

Rik is forty-one, mildly geeky and very clever. He could have made millions in Silicon Valley. He sees a problem, mulls it over in his head, comes up with a solution and then waits for everyone to catch up. In 2019 he was instrumental in installing the UCH electronic health record and wrote an app that now runs our working lives. Three years prior to that, in a week's 'holiday', he delivered twenty-four-hour electricity to a bush hospital in Kenya by taking out solar panels and an inverter and installing them on the roof. I went to Cornwall and put my head through the sail of someone else's windsurfer.

'Are you around Wednesday?' he asked.

'Yeah, sure.'

'We're gonna run some simulated scenarios. Can you come?'

'Of course.' Rik's mind was clearly on something else. 'Are you sure you're OK?'

'Yeah, yeah I'm just . . .' He paused. 'I'll see you Wednesday.'

That afternoon, still slightly shell-shocked, I returned to work as normal. At 2.30 p.m. the haematologist, bedside nurse and I sat down in the relatives' room to talk to Susan's family. Her haematologist recapped on the state of her disease and the lack of therapeutic options, and I went through all her vital systems that were failing,

'We've been doing all we can,' I explained, 'but she is still deteriorating and I think we have to accept that we have come to the end of the line. I am so sorry.'

They looked exhausted and devastated, but not surprised by anything we'd said. They'd always known that the chances of her getting out of ICU were slim, but she'd been determined to give it a go.

Once we'd finished, we paused and then asked if they had any questions. For a moment they looked silently at the floor, but then her husband looked up and cleared his throat.

'So what happens now?'

'First of all,' I began, 'we will make absolutely sure that she doesn't suffer.'

'Thank you.'

'And then we have a couple of options. We can leave things as they are or we can gently reduce some of the artificial support and let nature take its course.'

'Take the breathing tube out?'

'Not necessarily.'

'Can we spend some time with her?' Her daughter asked, 'before . . .'

'Of course. There's no rush, take as much time as you want.'

My next port of call was 'Resus' (short for Resuscitation) in the Emergency Department (ED) which was previously called Accident and Emergency and before that Casualty. (I don't know why they can't stick with a name, although my own department has been called, variously, the Intensive Care Unit, the Critical Care Unit and the Intensive Therapy Unit, so who am I to judge?) There was a possible ICU admission that I needed to review.

Resus is a five-bedded area for the sickest patients in the ED. It is a vibrant, noisy, messy place that sees all of life from six-month-olds with croup struggling to breathe, right through to ninety-year-olds who have been found unconscious on the floor of their homes. It's crowded, chaotic and stressful. Quite often all five patients look sick enough to warrant ICU admission.

Awaiting me that day was a seventy-five-year-old man with a viral exacerbation of his chronic obstructive pulmonary disease (he'd tested negative for Covid). He was extremely breathless, but the question was: should this man be admitted to ICU and ventilated?' He was certainly sick enough, he looked awful, but would it do him any good? He was already receiving support for each breath via a tight mask strapped to his face, but it wasn't enough. Should we limit the support there or should we put him to sleep, put a tube down his trachea and fully ventilate him? If we did, would we ever get him off the ventilator again, and even if we did, would we get him home to a quality of life he'd be happy with? He was still smoking, rarely left his home, breathless after ten yards walking on the flat and reliant on his family for shopping and most cooking. His function was already extremely limited, and weeks on ICU would only make him weaker. On the other hand, he enjoyed the racing on TV and visits from his mates, he just about looked after himself and he had never required ICU admission before. He was borderline, and the longer I do the job the more difficult I find these decisions. There is never much time, and the information is almost always incomplete. The easiest option in many ways is to ventilate everyone, but it's not always the right one, so the first thing to establish was what he wanted. Unsurprisingly he was too breathless and drowsy to tell me, so what did his family think? His son had dropped him off, but then he'd had to dash off to pick up his own kids, so had he put anything in writing about what treatments he would or would not want in these circumstances (an advanced directive)? Not that anyone could find.

I had to ventilate him, at least in the short term. If I didn't, he'd not long be for this world, and I didn't have enough information to make firm predictions about his eventual outcome.

As I trudged back up the three flights of stairs to the ICU I glanced at my watch. It was already 4.15 p.m. I still hadn't seen my poor man with pneumonia and I was meant to be starting the afternoon round to take over the south half of the unit from my colleague Alice.

Officially I am Alice's mentor, although from day one it's been a two-way street. She is diligent, generous and phenomenally effective. She is also a worrier, which is one of the reasons that we get on so well. Three years ago a rival London teaching hospital tried to poach her, offering her the world, and I had to mentor my socks off to persuade her to stay. Her interest is education, but rather than just deliver the odd lecture and teaching session like I do, she runs major sections of two training programmes and is adored by her trainee doctors. When she went on maternity leave last year, the positive feedback from our own ICU trainees plummeted.

She was waiting patiently for me at the main desk of ICU when I returned, so, having briefly worried together about Covid over a cup of tea, we set off around her patients. That afternoon the south side was generally under control. Alice had several patients making slow progress after prolonged periods of ventilation, a few more ready to go back to a normal ward (when beds became available), a patient she'd just put a tracheostomy in who was recovering from pancreatitis, the Covid patient (whom she'd already reviewed and was stable) and four 'post-ops' recently arrived. Four more were still expected. Only one patient was worryingly sick, but she'd put a robust plan in place, and I'd check on his progress later, before I went home. At 5.30 we'd seen them all, so I suggested Alice go home, but I knew she wouldn't. There were two sets of relatives she wanted to talk to and a trainee who wanted to bend her ear. She'd be there another hour at least, probably two.

By 7.30 p.m. I was weary and hungry. The ward round of my north side patients had taken longer than I'd planned, partly because of a referral from one of the wards and partly because every patient seemed to have relatives at the bedside who, quite reasonably, wanted an update. The patient with pneumonia I'd neglected was improving and extremely understanding about being missed out on the morning round, but Susan had deteriorated further. She was near the end now, but she looked peaceful and was surrounded by her family. We agreed I'd turn off the blood pressure drugs, but leave the breathing tube in place. I asked if they'd like us to call a priest or other religious leader.

'No, thank you,' her husband replied with a half chuckle. 'She'd be horrified!'

I sat on the bus on the way home staring out of the window and thinking about the lunchtime meeting. The government had by now warned of the potential for school closures and the banning of mass gatherings, and vulnerable people had been warned to shield. Those with coughs were being asked to self-isolate, but the rest of us were still going about our business, essentially as normal. Italy was now in lockdown, but we were still in 'mitigation'. It was 9 March. After that night I was due to be working in the operating theatre for two weeks. I wondered what the ICU would be like when I came back.

'Dad, Dad, Dad.' As I pushed the front door closed behind me, my son Tom swung from the banister and landed in the hallway with a thud. 'Guess what?'

'Hi Tom. How was school?'

'Fine, boring, but I've been invited to Jack's birthday. It's on Saturday at Flip Out, then McDonald's, and they want you to come too. There's twelve of us going, with his dad, who's really nice.'

Jack's dad is really nice, but it sounded hideous.

'Umm, great. Possibly. You can definitely go.'

' 'Sup, Dad.' Tom's twin sister Edie sauntered passed us, barely looking up from her phone.

'Hi, Edie, how was school.'

'It was OK. I'm going to have a shower.'

'Did you have that maths test?'

'Yeah. Mum's sculpting a horse's head.'

'OK, great.'

'She's got a commission.'

My wife Tish, an actress, has diversified more recently into garden design and sculpting. She often jokes about being a jack-of-all-trades, but her bronze sculptures are beautiful, although I have to admit that when Edie mentioned a 'horse's head' the infamous scene from *The Godfather* did flash through my mind.

I called in to work at eleven and was relieved to discover that one of our most sensible and senior registrars, Hannah, was on for the night shift. We discussed the post-operative cases who'd come in since I'd left, Alice's sick patient who was following the plan, the Covid patient who was busy on his phone and Susan, who had just passed away. Hannah told me about a young patient with a fluctuating conscious level that she had just seen on the ward, and we agreed that he should come down to us via the CT scanner. We talked about bed availability (we had three empty beds, including two side rooms, so plenty of wiggle room for the night), and I told her to phone me when she'd got the result of the scan. She called at 1 a.m. to say the CT was normal and that her money was on sub-clinical seizures (abnormal 'seizure' activity in the brain that manifests as unconsciousness rather than limb shaking), so she had loaded him with anti-epileptics and was about to do a lumbar puncture to check for meningitis or viral encephalitis. For the moment, however, he was stable.

'No temperature?' I asked.

'Low grade, and normal bloods, but we're going to start him on antibiotics and anti-virals just in case.'

'Sounds like a plan.'

I thanked her, hung up and rolled over. Within seconds I was fast asleep again. There is nothing like being on with a registrar that you trust.

She called again at 4 a.m. to let me know she was admitting a patient who was deeply unconscious after an overdose of the recreational drug GHB. He was intubated in the Emergency Department but otherwise stable and just needed time to sleep it off. Again I thanked her and briefly enquired about the other patient with the low conscious level. The lumbar puncture had been done, she said, but the results were not back yet, and there were no signs of ongoing seizures. If anything, he was a bit more alert.

The next thing I knew, it was 6.40 a.m., and my alarm was going off. It had been a quiet night – for me at least.

Over the next couple of days we drew up standard operating procedures (SOPs) and checklists for key Covid tasks. Every procedure we did would be different for Covid patients, partly because of the PPE and partly because we'd have to isolate these patients and everything they touched from everyone else. A massive re-education programme was required, devised by people with no experience of the disease and who were therefore making it up as they went along.

On the Wednesday (11 March) Rik, with some anaesthetic colleagues, tackled intubation. This is our core skill. Putting a patient to sleep and inserting a tube into their trachea to artificially ventilate them for an operation or a stay on ICU is on page one of the manual, but in Covid it would be more complicated. This was a high-risk procedure for the doctor, possibly the highest risk in terms of catching Covid. Not only were the patient and doctor going to be in very close proximity, mouths and noses within a few inches of each other, it was also an aerosol generating medical procedure (AGMP). At the time, Covid was thought to be spread by two routes: droplet and fomite. Either it was carried from one patient to the next directly by droplets of water in the breath or it settled on a surface (fomite) and was then picked up by a person's hand and subsequently transferred to their mouth, nose or eyes. Unlike measles, it was not thought to be airborne (able to linger in the air on tiny particles), so should not normally travel very far in the atmosphere. AGMPs, however, artificially manipulate the airway and the secretions within it (packed with virus), creating aerosols (small droplets of water), which could then transport the virus longer distances in high concentrations. If, as was thought likely, the inoculation dose related to the severity of infection, intubators would be right in the firing line. We needed to make our intubations as safe as possible for both the patient and the doctor. (Subsequently the boundary between droplet and airborne transmission has become blurred, and it appears that Covid can to an extent be transmitted on smaller particles and travel further in the air even in the absence of AGMPs).

At 2 p.m. twelve of us gathered in the antechamber of our isolation side room on the ICU (social distancing as much as we could). The aim was to run through the whole procedure as a simulation using a mannequin as the patient, from preparation to clear up, flushing out problems along the way. From this we would produce a 'Covid intubation checklist', a 'Covid intubation standard operating procedure (SOP)' and a training video (the simulation was being filmed). Rik and one of the anaesthetic consultants were up front, fully donned and playing the roles of intubators; an ICU nurse was their assistant, and two others played runners. There were two cameramen (one iPhone, one Samsung), one note-taker and four observer/commentators. I was at the back of the crowd, struggling to see or hear and keeping my mouth shut. There were plenty of opinions.

Every step of the process seemed to throw up a new list of problems. Who should go into the room and what equipment should they take? Once in, we wouldn't be able to come out again to grab something we'd forgotten, but anything we took into the room was then 'dirty', and would be thrown away or require decontamination. Which technique should we use? Should it be protocolized or at the individual doctor's discretion? What back-up equipment should be available? How and who should people call for help? Which drugs should we use?

It felt as if people were asking questions for the sake of it now, and my mind started to wander. I found myself glancing at the BBC website on my phone. The World Health Organization had just declared Covid a global pandemic, but despite alarming rates in Madrid, 3,000 Spanish football fans were on their way to the UK to watch Atlético Madrid play Liverpool. In the west of the country tens of thousands of people were crammed into the Cheltenham festival.

At the end of the meeting I'd meant to catch Rik to find out what had been bothering him two days before, but he seemed fine again and was caught up in a hive of activity, so I left him to it.

The next day, while others edited together the training video and wrote up the SOP and checklist, I returned to my normal theatre list of breast cancer patients. It felt odd to be doing elective surgery. These patients needed their operations and had just as much right to attention as Covid patients, but I was distracted and impatient. I felt restless, and guilty that I wasn't preparing for Covid – as if it was a big looming exam that I should be spending every waking hour revising for.

By now people were putting plans together for elective surgery to be scaled back and for the ICU to expand into the operating theatres, but still it all felt fragmented and ad hoc. One more Covid patient skirted through ICU and again did not need ventilation, but otherwise things continued to function as normal. There was a strong sense of anticipation, but for the most part, for the majority of people it was just that – waiting.

On Fridays I chair the weekly anaesthetic department academic meeting and that Friday (13 March) I cancelled the talk and devoted the meeting to a demonstration of PPE. I thought it would be a good chance for me to practise, so with Rik (who again seemed pensive and distracted) as my buddy I stood in front of seventy-five anaesthetists and donned and doffed. There was a strange atmosphere in the room, lots of laughter and heckling. I couldn't tell if people were genuinely relaxed and enjoying themselves or actually tense, but covering it up. My demonstration was pretty clumsy and inarticulate, so perhaps it was a simple choice between laugh or cry. As I was preparing the kit, I lectured the audience about the importance of hand hygiene and not touching their faces, only to lick my fingers in order to pull apart my plastic apron. My gaffe was met by a joyful screech of outrage from the front row and dozens of righteous pointy fingers.

At the end of the meeting the discussion turned to the subject of self-isolation. This was long before swab tests were available routinely for healthcare workers, and people were worried about bringing Covid to work and inadvertently spreading it around the hospital. Our clinical lead initially suggested that anyone with a sniffle should stay home to be on the safe side, but when I asked for a show of hands of all those with a sniffle, three-quarters of the audience raised their hands. Fever or a persistent cough would be required to get time off work.

On Saturday, 14 March I received a Whatsapp from Rik: 'We need a meeting, important. 8 p.m. tonight in the anaesthetic department. Please try to come or Zoom in.' The whole world was suddenly Zooming, even in the creaky old NHS.

By 8.05 p.m. on that Saturday night twenty of us were sitting in a semi-circle waiting to hear what he had to say. Another twenty were listening in online. Rik was worried. He'd listened to an Italian intensivist on a webinar and then talked to some modellers and come to the conclusion that our numbers were woeful underestimates. We were working on government figures, which suggested a doubling time for admissions of five days, but according to Rik's model, a figure of three days would be nearer the truth. He then put up a graph of what this would mean in terms of numbers if something radical wasn't done to flatten the curve, and it made for terrifying reading. We'd have slow growth for two weeks, reaching roughly thirty ICU patients by 28 March, but by 4 April we'd have eighty-three and a week after that, assuming the doubling rate continued, over 300. We had thirty-five ICU beds. If we filled every theatre with three patients and every space in recovery and used every ventilator of any description we might stretch to 130, but there'd be no more trained nurses or doctors, and we'd have run out of decent ventilators and filters long ago. At 300 it would be pandemonium. ICU patients would be everywhere; instead of ventilators we'd have medical students squeezing bags. We'd run out of drugs to keep people asleep, syringe drivers to deliver those drugs and quite possibly oxygen. It would be like a war zone.

By coincidence we'd admitted our first seriously sick Covid patient to ICU that day and were starting to put some solid plans in place, but outside life seemed to be going on as normal. Italy, France and Spain were all locked down, but our pubs, clubs and theatres were still open. The only advice about travel was for schools and those over seventy planning cruises, and there were no regular briefings, so there was little evidence that anything was being done to curb Rik's predictions – yet.

We needed to readjust and prepare for a super-surge of critically sick patients. It was terrifying, but nevertheless it felt like a turning point. This was serious, we needed to get organized, accelerate our plans and brace for the worst. The focus and cohesion in the room was palpable, and Rik had become our unofficial Covid leader.

That Monday we got to work. We trawled the literature and phoned colleagues in Italy and China to get as much clinical information as we could. Elective surgery was rapidly scaled back, we moved beds and equipment to form new makeshift ICUs, we rewrote the trainee rotas and began to draft in more doctors: ex-trainees, future trainees, trainees from other specialties with ICU experience, trainees from other specialities who'd like ICU experience, anyone willing to come and work with us. We also finalized our SOPs and checklists and trained as many people as possible in the new ways of working.

The anaesthetists were crucial. There were lots of them, they had the most relevant and transferable skills, and the closure of elective surgery would free them up, so at lunchtime I arranged to meet up with Jamie.

Jamie and I were appointed as consultants within a few months of each other – he claims to be younger but has never proved it. He is an anaesthetist and pain specialist who asked to be described as tall, dark and handsome. He was one of the team working out how the anaesthetists should be redeployed. He is also a great friend and along with his architect boyfriend Sammy was often to be found drinking wine in our kitchen late into the night before Covid. I found him in the anaesthetic office surrounded by pieces of paper covered with lists of names.

'Hey, how's it going?'

'Average,' he replied. He rarely admits to being better than average.

'Where have you been?'

'Wales.'

'Glamorous. Holiday?'

'Three weeks.'

'You've been in Wales for three weeks? From the end of February?'

'Yeah. We can't take Vuppe out of the country.'

'What's Vuppe?'

'Our new Cavapoochon. I told you.'

I looked at him blankly.

'Puppy, Jim.'

He thinks I am heartless because I don't coo over pictures of puppies.

'Oh yeah. How's it going?'

'Stressful. She didn't like Wales.'

'You do know there's a pandemic on?'

'Do you think she might get it?'

'Get what?'

'Covid.'

'Vuppe?'

'She's very sensitive.'

'Probably. Are you going to come and do ICU?'

'I'm allergic to ICU.'

'What does Vuppe even mean?'

'It's from *Rare Exports*, a horror film about a boy who is trying to kill Santa.'

'Nice. Why don't you bring her for a walk on the Heath?'

'She's not allowed outside yet. And I'm worried Betty might eat her.'

Betty is our Border terrier, who admittedly has a bad track record with small fluffy animals.

'We should talk anaesthetic rotas.'

'Yeah.' Jamie gestured to the piles of paper in front of him. 'Adi, Viki and James have already worked most of it out.'

'Thank God for that.'

UCH has ninety consultant anaesthetists and a further fifty trainees. Of the ninety, eight consultants have split jobs between anaesthesia and ICU like me, and even though they don't any more, the rest have all worked in ICU during their training. They might be rusty, but it is not an alien environment. ICU is a relatively recent invention. It originated in the polio epidemic of the 1950s, when that virus left thousands of people unable to breathe by destroying the nerves to their diaphragms. They lay in rows, some with just their heads protruding from the iron lungs that sucked the air into their paralysed bodies and others with medical students by their sides, squeezing bags to ventilate their lungs. The ICUs that subsequently sprang up around the UK through the 1970s and 1980s were run almost exclusively by anaesthetists. They already used ventilators and medications to manipulate the blood pressure for anaesthetized patients, and in the early days ICU was not dissimilar to a prolonged period in the operating theatre. It has moved on in the last forty years, but it was only in the early 2000s that it broke free and became its own specialty with a separate training programme and specialist qualification. Even now all anaesthetists spend at least six months of their training in ICU.

The anaesthetic department is usually the biggest in a hospital. Alongside the operating theatre, anaesthetists work in pain clinics, pre-assessment clinics, endoscopy, bronchoscopy, ICU, radiotherapy, brachytherapy, CT, MRI, interventional radiology, ED, labour wards and the surgical wards on pain rounds. There are few departments they don't support in one way or another. Over the next week the vast majority of that work would disappear. They'd continue to run an emergency theatre, anaesthetize for some cancer surgery at Westmoreland Street, and babies would continue to be born, but otherwise everything would be stopped. All surgery that could wait was put on hold: hip replacements, tonsillectomies, prostate surgery, hernias, hysterectomies, even some cancer surgery. Many procedures such as endoscopies and bone marrow transplants were also postponed, and just as worryingly, investigations slowed right down, potentially delaying time-sensitive cancer diagnoses. Pre-assessment clinics were no longer required, and to a large extent, thanks to the fear of Covid, people stopped coming into the Emergency Department. The anaesthetists would need to completely change their working lives and focus on the effort to fight Covid.

Anaesthesia is an unusual area of medicine. The better we are at doing the job, the more invisible we become. We are not the ones who make people better in the operating theatre, but we can make them a lot worse, and it is often quoted that 50 per cent of the country still believe we are not doctors. However, when it all goes badly wrong in hospital it is the anaesthetists that people call. We are the ones who can rescue the airway, take over the breathing and support the circulation – keep you alive in other words. Through the pandemic, the tribe of 11,000 or so anaesthetists around the country would be vital to the Covid response, and so it was at UCH. Over fifty (roughly half consultants, half trainees) were redeployed full-time to ICU, and the rest formed teams and worked twelve-hour shifts, day and night: a transfer team, an intubation team, an obstetric team, an emergency team and a Westmoreland team. Jamie assigned himself to the emergency team, or 'family', as he insisted on calling it.

The anaesthetists also, along with operating department staff and senior ICU nurses, converted the operating theatres complex into an ICU. They replaced trolleys with beds, reconfigured the electronic health record on the local computers, sourced monitors, disposables, infusion pumps, drugs, anaesthetic machine ventilators, PPE and walkie-talkies. The post-operative recovery room, the holding bay and eight operating theatres became the ICU bed areas, the theatre reception a PPE donning and doffing station, the surgeons' tearoom a storeroom and the outside corridor a communication hub. I remember walking around theatres, now known as 'the Pods', the day before the first patient was admitted. It was unrecognizable. They'd created a fully functioning twenty-bedded ICU in a week. Within another week it would be forty-four beds, then fifty-five. Creating one ICU bed usually takes weeks of planning, a feasibility study and input from multiple departments. This group created fifty-five beds in two weeks, on their own. It was an extraordinary achievement.

Finally Alice and I sat down to work out how the ICU

consultants would work. Like ICU nurses, we were a fixed resource, and if the ICU was going to quadruple in size, we needed a serious rethink. The ICU ward round, trouble-shooting acute deteriorations and decision-making about the appropriateness of ICU therapies are our unique skills, our bread and butter. We do these things every day, and it would be unfair to expect others, who don't, to step in. I spent six months of my anaesthetic training at Great Ormond Street Hospital (GOSH). At the end of that period I would have happily anaesthetized any number of six-month-old babies, but leave me with one now and within minutes I'd be curled up in a ball, weeping and begging for someone to take over. Likewise, it would be wrong to ask a paediatric anaesthetist to run the ICU.

There were eighteen ICU consultants, and initially everyone stepped forward. All offered to go on to whatever rota we pro-duced, but we had misgivings from the start. Some were vulnerable in terms of their own health, and several were in their sixties. Should they be going on to night shifts and sur-rounding themselves with Covid patients? They insisted they should, but before we even started the three causing us most concern all caught Covid outside the hospital and were signifi-cantly ill. Despite the dwindling numbers, we wrote a full-time, rolling, nine-week rota with thirteen-hour shifts and resident nights for eighteen consultants. Initially a few of us did extra shifts to cover the shortfall, but fortunately David had already put out an urgent advert for more consultants. Within two weeks he'd interviewed three favourable candidates and wel-comed them to their new consultant posts. We were back up to full complement.

The next day Rik caught me in the office.

'Ah, Jim, got a job for you.'

'OK,' I replied hesitantly, praying it wasn't anything to do with equipment or computers.

'You'll like it.' he continued. 'Ethics.'

'Right,' I replied, both relieved and confused.

'You've got an interest, haven't you?'

Have I? I thought. I'm a fan of the Radio 4's *Moral Maze*, but my interest certainly doesn't stretch to a qualification or even a course. I'd hope that all doctors have at least the level of interest I do, but then I remembered I had been bleating on about moral luck a lot recently, and the ethics of advanced directives.

'Suppose so,' I shrugged.

'Great.'

I saw Rik mentally tick off another job in his mind as he made for the door.

'One thing,' I added, hoping to cement my ethical credentials. 'I think we should set up a three wise people system, for all major and controversial decisions.'

'Agreed,' he replied, 'and we should have a Trust Ethics Group or committee. Oh, and can you keep on top of any national documents?'

'Yup,' I promised, weakly, and he was gone.

The ethics of ICU are difficult at the best of times. Whenever an expensive new drug is brought to market, the National Institute of Clinical Excellence (NICE) assesses it. They decide whether it is cost-effective, whether the improvement to the quality or duration of patients' lives is worth the cost. It is a tough, but necessary process. A drug that costs £10,000 a shot and lengthens life by a matter of days is not a good use of taxpayers' money, but NICE have never assessed ICU. The cost of a day on ICU is approximately £1,700. What benefit does that need to reap to be cost-effective?

We often talk about a reasonable chance of return to a meaningful quality of life, but what is a meaningful quality of life? For some people life itself is sacred, just being alive even if deeply and irreversibly unconscious. For others a certain level of disability or pain makes life not worth living. And what is a reasonable chance? 1 per cent, 5 per cent, 20 per cent? Do the two – chance and quality of life – multiply together? Is 30 per cent chance of 70 per cent quality equal to 70 per cent chance of 30 per cent quality? And who decides? The patients are usually unconscious, so the doctors? The family?

Our ultimate responsibility is to seek consent when a patient has capacity, act in their best interests when they don't and not offer futile therapies. This is broadly the ethics of fairness. Every patient should be treated fairly, whatever their age, race, creed, gender, sexuality, etc. and in normal times this works. The boundaries get blurred in busy winters when beds become sparse and high-risk surgery gets postponed, but we can usually find a bed somewhere if someone really needs it. In a pandemic, however, when resource limitation becomes an issue (be it equipment or staff), the ethics of benefit begin to enter the equation. How much benefit will this patient get from this treatment and what are the chances of that benefit? A twenty-year-old might benefit more than a seventy-year-old because they have more potential years of life, but if the seventy-year-old has an 80 per cent chance of recovery and the twenty-year-old only 20 per cent, it becomes more complicated.

I was beginning to wish I'd been given something to do with equipment or computers.

Luckily for me, the three wise people concept was a tried and trusted one. For a single clinician difficult ethical decisions over matters of life and death can be a huge burden, and sense checking with a colleague or two is standard practice. The change I planned for Covid times was to make this a formal, mandatory process. The decisions could be divided into two categories: which therapies should be offered, what we call a Treatment Escalation Plan (TEP) and for how long those treatments should be continued. These are often referred to as withhold and withdrawal decisions, and we wrestle with them in normal times, but with Covid there might be three crucial differences.

The first was the number of patients. The sheer volume of critically ill people meant that we might be making far more of these decisions than normal. That rang alarm bells, about both the quality of the decision-making and the potential moral injury to those deciding.

The second was that this was a new disease. All our usual parameters, our knowledge base, were on shifting sands. We'd never treated anyone with Covid before, so how could we be sure that the usual rules applied?

The final difference was the time frame. Decisions about withdrawal of care can take a long time to enact. When we have decided that ongoing treatment is futile, we discuss it with the family or advocates of the patient. Usually they agree or accept our judgement, but not uncommonly they have doubts, or even disagree. Often after a few more meetings we are all on the same page, but sometimes they request second opinions and, rarely, refuse to accept our decision and consider legal advice. In my fifteen years as an ICU consultant we have never had a case go to court, but the process of consensus can take days, weeks even. In Covid times, with the pressure on resources, we might not be able to allow these decisions to take days or weeks. Put bluntly, we might need the bed for the next patient.

I assembled a small group of ICU colleagues, called some key players from other specialties and booked our first Trust Ethics Group meeting for the next week. The following day I received an email from the chief executive formally requesting I become Trust Ethics lead, and the same day Jon, a palliative care colleague, suggested I contact Baroness Julia Neuberger (chair of the hospital) to see if she'd chair a Clinical Ethics Advisory Group. This would be a much grander and more formal committee made up of clinicians, judges, religious leaders, academics and lay representatives, to offer advice, guidance and support for clinicians. I'd never met Baroness Neuberger, but I emailed her, and within half an hour she'd agreed.

By now I was suffering from what I have subsequently discovered to be anticipation fatigue. We had been working hard, preparing in huddles, discussing endlessly what might or might not happen, practising, training, and reorganizing, but I was still yet to don PPE for an actual Covid patient. The longer I waited, the more of an issue it became, and so when I was reassigned from theatre to ICU on 18 March, I was relieved as well as nervous.

It took me fifteen minutes to don the first time. My hands were sweaty, the tapes wouldn't stick, and I kept having to refer back to the crib sheet on the wall to check that I was putting it on right. Eventually, with the mask, first gloves, hat, gown, second gloves, tape, visor and apron safely on, I pushed open the door to a bay full of Covid patients.

It felt as if a weight had been lifted.

For a moment I stood and surveyed the scene. The PPE made me feel as if I was in my own bubble, cut off slightly from the world. Sounds were muffled, and seeing everything through a visor gave a sense of separation. It was a familiar scene in many ways – I have worked in that ICU bay for fifteen years – but also completely alien. The staff looked so different, each transformed into a different-sized version of the same thing – hat, visor, mask, apron and below-knee baggy blue gown. I couldn't tell who was who, or even which job each of them was doing. Was that a nurse or a physio or a junior doctor by bed 34? The patients were not in PPE, of course, because they already had Covid, but that just seemed to exaggerate the difference between the sick and the healthy. While the staff strode around the ward in full protective armour, the patients lay in flimsy backless gowns, powerless and vulnerable in their beds.

Some staff had their names and job titles scrawled across their aprons, and as I shuffled around the bay working out who was who, it struck me.

They were all just getting on with it.

They were hampered by the PPE, and everything looked awkward, but the nurses, physios and doctors were being as professional, gentle and busy as ever. They'd accepted the situation, taken it in their stride and carried on.

For some reason, whenever I put on an FFP3 mask my natural reaction is to breathe through my mouth. One edge of the mask fits over the nose, with a metal band to pinch into the nostrils and the other under the chin. I was never quite sure about the seal under my chin and I found myself opening my mouth subconsciously to pull the mask tighter. I was just wondering whether I did actually have an adequate seal or should go and re-don, when Viola, a staff nurse, approached.

'Do you want me to continue the deep sedation in bed 34? He was turned on to his back an hour ago, and his oxygen requirement has gone up to 70 per cent.'

'Yes,' I replied. My voice sounded strange and muffled even to me, and I couldn't quite tell if I was shouting at her or inaudible. 'We'll re-prone tonight. Let's keep him deep for today.'

'Great,' she bellowed back, her eyes smiling. I was shouting.

But I was up and running and I felt the tension drain away as I set about assessing the patients. I'd been scared of entering a bay full of Covid patients, but now I was here among the team in full protective gear, I felt safe, probably safer than in a shop or on the tube. By now (18 March) I'd stopped using public transport and going to crowded spaces like the cinema and the pub. I was even giving people a wide birth on the pavement and yet in this room, full of some of the sickest Covid patients in the country, I was fine.

Over the next few days I felt energized. I was on the shop

floor, doing the job I'd trained for, part of a team, and it felt good, exciting even. The patients seemed to be responding to our treatments. Some of them were very sick, intubated and ventilated, but others were awake, breathing comfortably on tight-fitting CPAP masks.

CPAP – or Continuous Positive Airway Pressure – is equivalent to opening your mouth and sticking your head out of the roof of a car that's travelling at 70 miles per hour. Delivered via a sealed hood or a tight-fitting mask, it applies constant positive pressure to the lungs of awake patients. The aim is to open up collapsed air spaces and so improve oxygen uptake into the circulation, without having to put the patient to sleep, intubate them and put them on a ventilator.

Some patients on CPAP were stuck, reliant for days on the postive pressure and extra oxygen, but several turned around quickly and were soon on their way back to the ward. I remember thinking: *we can do this*. The nurses, doctors, physios, ward clerks – everyone has stepped up. If anyone can cope with this we can.

2. Lockdown

Boris Johnson announced lockdown on 23 March. The brakes were now on, but even if they were effective, we could not expect to see the impact for at least two more weeks. In the meantime, the patients would continue to flood in, so the government was encouraging hospitals to discharge as many inpatients home or into care homes as possible to make room.

One patient in particular personified those early shifts. John was a forty-one-year-old publican. He was cheerful and easygoing with no chronic health problems, but he was obese, weighing over 25 stones. From the start he'd required the CPAP mask and high amounts of oxygen. When I met him he was breathing 90 per cent oxygen.

The combination of 25 stones weight and 90 per cent oxygen via a CPAP mask causes me (and all but the coolest of my colleagues) to feel edgy. Obese patients store less oxygen in their lungs (because of upward compression by the abdomen) and, because of their high metabolic rate, they use up that oxygen more quickly. This, added to the fact that their airways are often more difficult to manage, makes for a double threat.

When we anaesthetize a patient (for an operation or to be put on a ventilator in intensive care) we give them 100 per cent oxygen for three or four minutes beforehand. This means that all the nitrogen in their lungs is replaced with oxygen, giving them a two to three litre reservoir to be absorbed before they turn blue. It buys us some time (roughly five minutes in a slim, well patient). We then put the patient to sleep, paralyse them and take over their breathing by holding a tight mask to the face and squeezing a bag. Two minutes later, when the paralysis has had time to fully work, we insert a tube into their trachea (intubation) and attach that to a ventilator.

In the vast majority of cases this is straightforward; ventilating via a bag and mask is easy, and by using a laryngoscope (a four-inch handle attached to a curved metal blade with a light at the end, which slips down behind the tongue to allow us a view of the vocal cords) we can see exactly where to place the tube. We have plenty of time, and everyone is calm and composed. Certain conditions, however, alter that dynamic.

Some people are difficult or impossible to ventilate via a mask, some are difficult to intubate and some go blue much, much more quickly. John, at 25 stones and already on 90 per cent oxygen, had the potential to be all three. His lungs were already filled with almost as much oxygen as is possible and still, because of the damage to his lung tissue, he was barely getting enough through to his blood. There was no reserve. If we were we unable to ventilate him, his blood oxygen levels would plummet, and within a couple of minutes the lack of oxygen would cause his heart to slow and then stop. He might well be difficult to ventilate via a mask (there was no way of knowing until we tried), and intubation might not be straightforward. If all else failed, the final step of the algorithm would be to make a hole in the front of John's neck and insert a tube that way, but in his case, by that stage, the situation would probably be beyond salvaging.

Normally, when people require more than about 60 per cent oxygen via a CPAP mask we start to get nervous. We consider putting them to sleep, intubating and taking over. Usually they have started to feel tired, increasingly breathless, agitated or all three, but John had been sitting comfortably on 90 per cent oxygen via a tight-fitting mask for days.

I was torn. If we were going to intubate, we should do it in daylight, in a controlled fashion, using the most experienced team possible, and his oxygen parameters certainly suggested that he needed intubation. On three separate occasions I called the intubation team, resigned to the fact we should bite the bullet and put a tube down. On one occasion we even got as far as donning PPE and preparing our equipment, but when we looked into the room, he was sitting comfortably, listening to music and texting his family. We couldn't bring ourselves to intubate a man who looked so comfortable, however much oxygen he was needing, so we doffed and, with some trepidation, continued to watch and wait.

This phenomenon of 'happy hypoxia' was one we'd see over and over again. Patients who should have been gasping for air by all normal parameters weren't. People arrived at routine outpatient appointments feeling fine, only to be sent directly to the Emergency Department because of life-threateningly low oxygen levels, and John on his CPAP was similar. We were telling him he was at death's door, and he was telling us he was doing OK.

I finally felt confident that John would not require intubation on 24 March. When I saw him on the ward round that morning, he had definitively turned the corner. His oxygen requirements were down, his blood markers were improving, and he was able to sit himself out in the chair without assistance. It felt like a victory. We had done the right thing by listening to him, and he had got better. Two hours later on 24 March I was called back in to see Adam, the twenty-eight-year-old. His temperature was 41.8°C, and his blood pressure had crashed.

Adam was dark-haired, of average build, and two months previously he'd been fit and well, a painter and decorator in his dad's family business. For the last four weeks, however, he'd been suffering with fevers, a productive cough and breathlessness. Despite a course of antibiotics from his GP, his breathing had deteriorated, and on 17 March he'd come to hospital. He'd had no known contact with Covid and he hadn't been to any high-risk countries, but he had the classic combination of low lymphocytes (a white blood cell for fighting infection), high temperature and shadowing in both lungs on his chest x-ray. He tested positive for Covid and came straight to intensive care.

By the next day he had become too breathless, exhausted and agitated to carry on breathing on his own, so we'd put him to sleep, intubated him, and attached him to a state-of-the-art ICU ventilator. We then adjusted the settings to minimize the injury to his lungs and waited.

For a few days all seemed well. He was sick, but manageable. His blood markers of inflammation were impressively high, but they go up with infection and, as far as we understood, this was just a trait of Covid. Bide our time, we thought, look after the details, and when he was ready, he'd improve. At that point we'd gently wake him up, wean him off the ventilator, take the breathing tube out and send him on his way.

But his blood markers of inflammation didn't settle. They climbed further.

Inflammation is the body's response to infection, trauma or toxins. It is a complex system of white blood cells and molecules that interact to clear infections and repair damaged tissue. It must differentiate between foreign matter to be destroyed and the body's own cells to be left alone. Part of the system is innate. It will fight any foreign invader, but it can also adapt to remember previously encountered infections and kill them before they cause damage – immunity. Different infections require different responses and deficiency of a particular element of the process leaves us vulnerable to specific bugs. It is a finely tuned system. The red, hot swelling of a burn or an infected wound is inflammation. If that is happening in a vital organ such as the lungs, the performance of that organ is compromised, so there is a constant balance between inflammation – required to fight infection – and anti-inflammation – needed to protect the body's own vital functions. An overactive inflammatory system can cause as much trouble as an underactive one.

In ICU, we have been grappling with inflammation for forty years. Many of our patients are damaged first by infection and then by the body's response to that infection. Rather than kill off the infection locally and allow the patient to heal, the inflammation runs wild throughout the body and knocks out one system after another. The temperature and the pulse rise, and if it's really severe the blood pressure falls. The whole patient becomes a red, hot, swollen, infected wound. Again this is usually time-limited and a necessary evil, but the human body can only put up with so much.

We have attempted to meddle with the inflammatory process many times, knocked out this bit or bolstered that bit, but in ICU it has never really worked. Killing the bugs with antibiotics and anti-virals is often effective if you get there quickly enough, but there have been no other magic bullets.

Over the subsequent days it became clear that Adam's body was highly inflamed. We had drugs that could target different molecules of inflammation with pinpoint accuracy and stop them in their tracks, but the problem was which molecule to aim for and when. If we stopped a particular process would it dampen the inflammation and allow him to recover or strip him of his defences and let the virus run wild?

There was no way of knowing, so we decided to change Adam's antibiotics and continued the supportive care. His blood markers were high, but his organ function was still relatively stable.

The previous night, however, Adam had taken a significant turn for the worse and not in the way that we'd expected. It wasn't just his lungs that had deteriorated, it was everything. His temperature shot up, his blood pressure dropped, his heart rate climbed, and his kidneys began to fail. Covid was meant to be a single-system disease, an inflammation of the lungs, but this man was shutting down, all of him, and he wasn't seventy with lots of chronic health problems. He was twenty-eight with none.

Overnight we had managed to control the situation to a certain extent. We'd cooled him, given fluids and drugs to bolster the blood pressure, turned him on to his front for his lungs and, realizing that things were still going in the wrong direction, given a dose of a powerful anti-inflammatory. For twelve hours all had seemed under control. His observations improved, and his temperature settled, but by the morning his fever was back, and his kidneys had turned off completely.

Having seen Adam on the morning ward round and set up a plan, I'd left the registrar and nurses at his bedside to put in an extra line and set him up on a kidney machine – 'the filter'.

By the time I got back into the bay, two nurses, an ICU registrar and a consultant anaesthetist were already around Adam's bed, their names and professions scrawled across their aprons in marker pen.

'Hi,' I said, glancing up at the monitor.

'Jimbo!' The consultant anaesthetist, another Jim and good friend, had just popped in to help transfer a patient. I've never seen him look so pleased to see me.

'Tell me.'

The registrar, who'd been injecting something into the line in Adam's neck, looked up.

'We'd got the vascath in and were just about to start him on the filter when his blood pressure crashed and his heart rate shot up to 160.'

The filter is the ICU equivalent of a dialysis machine. It

requires a large, two channel intravenous line (a 'vascath') to be positioned in one of the large veins of the groin or neck. The filter then sucks blood continuously out through one channel, washes out the waste products and then returns it through the other. It needs a stable blood pressure to run successfully.

'His temperature's still above 40,' added Chryso, one of the staff nurses.

'OK, lets dunk another sheet under the cold tap and wrap him in it. Have you been irrigating his bladder?' I looked back at the monitor. 'What rhythm is that?'

'Just Sinus tachy, I think.'

'And you've tried more fluid?'

'A litre, but he's still needing a massive dose of noradrenaline to keep his blood pressure up.'

'OK, thanks. Have you got a blood gas?'

'Yup, hang on.'

Chryso grabbed a piece of paper from the trolley next to her and handed it to me as she continued to run through another intravenous drip.

'Bloody hell!'

Adam's potassium was life-threateningly high now, and his blood profoundly acidic.

'OK.' I looked around my colleagues. Some continued to draw up drugs and run through lines, but the two junior doctors and one nurse had turned to me expectantly, 'We need to control the potassium with insulin and—'

'I'm drawing it up now.'

I nodded.

'Great, thanks.'

Rik and another consultant intensivist, Dave Brealey, joined us as the conversation jumped around the bed, a mixture of questions, answers, observations and suggestions.

'And can we get some calcium?'

'Already in.'

'And some sodium bicarbonate?'

'OK.'

'We have got to get his pressure up so we can start him on the filter,' I added, desperately.

The filter would clear the acid and potassium more permanently and so improve the environment for the heart and other organs to function.

'We've tried, it clotted,' came the immediate reply.

'Can we try again?'

Dave Brealey is my contemporary and was nicknamed 'Tigger' as a trainee. He has boundless energy and is a naturally gifted intensivist. There's no one I would have preferred to be alongside me at that moment. He was above Adam's head now, fiddling with the Doppler probe going through his mouth into his gullet to measure the blood flow out of the heart.

'Let's try a small dose of beta blocker,' he suggested, 'very gently to slow his heart rate down to, say, 120.'

'Yup.' I nodded. If we slowed the heart, it might beat more effectively.

Rik put the echocardiogram probe on to Adam's chest wall, and we watched his heart pounding away as best it could, but it was already failing.

We were all working as efficiently as we could, but the PPE made everything more difficult. The area around Adam's bed was crowded with machines, equipment and people shuffling awkwardly past each other in bulky gowns. Occasionally an alarm from one of the other three patients in the bay distracted a nurse's attention for a moment, but apart from that all the focus was on Adam. It was hot, stuffy and noisy. Our voices were muffled through the masks, so every request or question had to be half shouted and often repeated. Three pairs of gloves meant that even a simple task, like putting in an intravenous line, was cumbersome and awkward. My visor was tight, and the mask was now pinching the bridge of my nose, but I couldn't adjust them. My gloves were covered with Covid. Touch my face and I'd catch it.

I was frustrated and I could hear the edge creeping into my voice. This was my patient, my responsibility. I've dealt with hundreds of medical emergencies in my career, countless cardiac arrests and near arrests. It is always chaotic and noisy, but this was different. He was young and previously fit and well. This was a new disease, and it was not what I'd been expecting.

Over the next ninety minutes we tried everything we could think of. We gave fluids and drugs to increase the blood pressure, other drugs to make the heart pump harder and others still to slow it down. Each one had benefits and side effects – cure one problem and you almost inevitably made another worse. We gave sodium bicarbonate to neutralize the acid in the blood, sugar and insulin to lower the potassium, calcium to stabilize the heart, and then we connected him to the filter to try to maintain the homeostasis. We wrapped him in wet towels and irrigated his bladder with cold water to bring down the temperature. All the while we were keeping a watchful eye to ensure that he was fully sedated and unaware.

For short periods we were winning. We got his temperature down, then his heart rate, and he seemed to improve. At one point Dave wrapped a cold, wet towel tight around Adam's head, and the heart rate fell by forty beats per minute, but it didn't last. Within minutes everything had crashed again, and we were pushing in huge doses of adrenaline to keep his heart pumping. People passed fluids, equipment, machines, samples and blood results back and forth through the door to the bay, communicating with the outside world by a combination of walkie-talkies and shouting. We verbalized everything; all our ideas, theories, requests, anxieties – everything, desperately searching for something that might turn it around, but gradually the periods of stability and hope became shorter. I looked under the sheets and saw the ominous patchwork of purple mottling creeping up his thighs and on to his abdomen. His tissues were dying.

At some point during the process Adam's mother arrived in the hospital. The nurses helped her into full PPE, brought her into the bay, and she walked tentatively over to the bed space to look down at her son. She saw his exposed torso, the breathing tube coming out of his mouth, the lines carrying his blood to and from the filter, the drug ampoules, the crumpled wet sheets, the crash trolley with drawers open and equipment spilling out, the fluids, the catheter, the syringes and torn packaging discarded around the bed, the machines and monitors and the eight of us surrounding him in our PPE. We paused for a second, then carried on, and she watched. Eventually she backed away to a seat by the door and listened to our efforts. Half an hour later, when I assume she couldn't bear it any more, she left.

Dave looked up at me from the head of the bed. I knew immediately what he was thinking. The blood pressure was down to forty again, and ominously now the heart was slowing too: eighty, seventy, fifty. The sharp spikes on the ECG had broadened. 'Agonal' we call it, and it means only one thing. Every four or five beats there was a pause, then another weak, flick of pulse on the blood pressure trace. He was dying. There was nothing more we could do.

'OK,' I said, looking round the eight shattered faces, 'I think we should stop. Anyone disagree?' A part of me was desperate for someone to disagree, but no one did. We watched as his heart twitched for a few more seconds and then stopped.

'Thank you, everyone, I'll go and find his family.'

I threw my mask in the bin, washed my hands and trudged back down the corridor. I felt desperate. What had happened?

Had I missed something? Should we have tried a novel anti-inflammatory sooner? He was the first patient I'd seen die of Covid and he was twenty-eight years old.

I pushed open the door to the relatives' room, shuffled in and perched against a bin. Four faces stared up at me.

They knew.

'Hello,' I began, 'My name is Jim, I'm one of the intensive care consultants. You're all Adam's family?'

'Brother.'

'That's his mum,'

'Sister.'

'Father.'

I nodded back to each in turn.

'I am so sorry.'

His mother's jaw tightened as she nodded slowly, and her family wrapped her in all the support and love they could.

I don't remember the rest of the conversation. I remember they were calm, despite being desperately upset, and I am sure they asked questions that I couldn't really answer. Like so many families at these terrible moments, they also said thank you.

I hope that being in the room when we were trying to resuscitate Adam helped his mother somehow. I believe at least she knows that we did all we could, but I am also aware that that's scant comfort.

I have never got used to breaking bad news to relatives. Walking into a room full of people you've never met to tell them the worst news they'll ever hear feels so wrong. It should be done by someone that they know and trust. Watching a face collapse with the horror of what you are saying is awful. I used to work hard to control my emotions and stay professional, I thought that was what was required, but I don't any more. I can't. I don't know what's right or wrong. Mostly families seem pleased to see that we are human, that we care, but occasionally it feels intrusive and voyeuristic to be present any longer than necessary at such a raw and personal moment.

What has become clear to me is that even at the lowest point, people are capable of the most incredible humanity and dignity.

That evening I went over and over the case in my mind trying to think of things I could have done differently. I pictured his mother back at home in Camden trying to make sense of it all. Her son had been fit and well. Why him? He was the youngest reported Covid death in the country at the time, the first under thirty. I wondered how many more there would be like him and what we should do differently next time. One of the hospital's communication team telephoned me to ask for an outline of the case. There would almost certainly be press interest. As I told her about Adam, the anxiety bubbled up again. I spoke to Rik and Dave and suggested we set up a meeting to discuss our strategy for the next 'Adam'. They were shaken by what had happened but at the same time convinced we'd done everything possible for him. They agreed that a meeting would be a good idea.

When I got home, I kissed Tom and Edie goodnight, listened to their plans for home schooling (scanty at best) and sat down with Tish. I wasn't much company. We talked about the kids, about lockdown and eventually about Adam. I often come home worried or upset about a patient, and invariably Tish makes me feel better. She listens, she asks questions, she sympathizes, and we move on, but that night I couldn't.

If Covid could kill Adam, it could kill any of us.

3. Nightingale

31 March 2020

'What . . . if it doesn't work?'

'Doesn't work?' Our guide looked up at me.

'The model . . .' I stopped and glanced around the eight faces staring back at me, waiting. I hate conflict, but I can't stop myself.

We were standing at the far east end of the Excel Centre, halfway down a corridor of forty-two ICU cubicles. Behind us was another corridor, and another, and another, all the way back down the 600 metre hall; creating up to 2,000 ICU beds in this, the South Hall, with another 2,000 to follow in the North Hall opposite. The size of it was barely comprehensible. This row was solid, fully built, as was the one behind, but beyond that the bed spaces seemed less and less distinct, blurring into each other like the crowd scene of a movie.

Up close, the cubicles reminded me of stands at a trade fair, each white, 16 metres square and open fronted. One was fully kitted out with electricity, pipelines, a bed, a ventilator, infusion pumps, suction and a trolley of equipment. The 'show' cubicle of the Nightingale Hospital, London.

Our guide smiled.

'Then we'll have to be honest and to rethink. We've got to be willing to learn, always.'

It was an impressive display of restraint, by her. I felt awful.

While Rik was scaring us with his case-doubling rates back at UCH, the head of the ICU response to Covid for North Central

London was grappling with the same problem on a much bigger scale. He'd quickly calculated that we'd need not just to double our ICU bed capacity across the sector, but to quadruple it – or more. Multiplying up for the whole of London, that would mean 2,000 extra ICU beds, a number that quickly became 4,000. I don't know the details of the calculations, but I do know that lots of clever people were modelling it and agreed: it was a real possibility. The team leading the ICU response for London had to find a solution – in days.

They could have tried to create this capacity within existing hospitals. They could have told hospitals to squeeze extra ICU beds into every possible nook and cranny, but they decided that this was not the best option. They came to the conclusion that the 'estate' of most hospitals could not accommodate such a sudden, massive expansion of ICU beds. In some hospitals this was because the oxygen supply was inadequate, in others equipment was the limiting factor, in others space, but for whatever reason all hospitals would reach their limit well before the required bed expansion.

They were also worried about efficiency. There are only so many trained ICU nurses in London and splitting them up to run three beds in the corner of one ward and four in an operating theatre somewhere else would be ICU-nurse 'hungry'. Each separate area would need a minimum number of trained nurses, so the smaller the areas, the less efficient the system. The solution, they decided, was 'barn ventilation'.

The idea was that they would set up a huge area, a 'barn', filled with ventilated patients. The barn would be divided into 'Nightingale'-style wards consisting of two rows of twenty-one beds facing each other (based on the layout developed by Florence Nightingale). The design meant that staff could keep an eye on several patients at once and move easily from bed to bed to carry out the necessary care.

National guidelines suggest that in normal times one ICU consultant, along with a junior doctor or two, should manage up to fifteen ICU patients. There should be one nurse per bed space and adequate input from allied healthcare professionals (physiotherapists, pharmacists, dieticians, etc.). The model for the Nightingale Hospital was that one ICU consultant would manage forty-two patients, with the support of doctors from other specialties, a senior nurse per ward, one trained ICU nurse per six patients and teams of other ward nurses and helpers. The work would be task orientated, with each shift run by a close-knit team, ideally recruited from a single hospital. All members of the team would follow the same twelve-hour shift patterns, always working together to optimize the bonding and team-work. They would deliver heavily protocolized care to simplify treatments and minimize errors.

The theory was that the new style of working, along with the Nightingale ward design, would make up for the reduced trained-staff-to-patient ratio. It was bold and innovative, but to succeed the protocolized care needed to work for the patient group, so they drew up strict admission criteria. Patients must be adults, previously fairly robust, sedated, intubated and venti-lated, not morbidly obese and with all their other systems (heart, kidneys, etc.) working, essentially, unsupported.

They then considered an exhaustive list of challenges and requirements: support services (labs, radiology, endoscopy, surgeons), staff services, the spiritual needs of staff, patients and relatives, transport, oxygen . . . The list went on, and for each they found a solution, all to be up and running in two weeks. It was logical, ambitious and impressive, but I had mis-givings.

I first heard mention of the Nightingale Hospital by chance, walking through the back of a Zoom call in our office on 20 March.

'We are talking to the intensivists,' a voice said from the computer. 'We know this is an ICU project.'

I smiled at my colleague, Tim, who was on the call. I didn't know what they were talking about, but I remember thinking, 'That's nice,' as I grabbed a coffee and headed back to the ICU.

Three days later the ICU matron, Elaine, took me aside.

'I don't know what to do,' she whispered, looking furtively over my shoulder.

'OK,' I replied.

'I've been asked to be a senior nurse in the new Nightingale Hospital at Excel.'

My heart sank. I have known Elaine for twenty years, and she epitomizes everything that is good about the NHS. Arguably my greatest achievement in my short tenure as clinical director between 2008 and 2012 was to persuade Elaine (and her friend Debbie) to apply jointly for the role of ICU matron. The nursing leadership was going through a difficult period at the time. Several ICU matrons had left in quick succession, vacancy and sickness rates were high (a sure sign of an unhappy unit), and some markers of care such as pressure area damage and MRSA infections were creeping in the wrong direction. Initially Elaine and Debbie were reluctant. It was a daunting proposition. Elaine had a young daughter and lived in Cambridgeshire, while Debbie was flying back home to see her dad in Ireland as often as she could. So I promised them that we'd be in it together, that I was appointing some great new consultants and that it would be 'fun, and an adventure'.

Eventually they acquiesced. I did appoint some great new consultants and for a year or so we were all in it together. We even had some fun, but soon the adventure was over for Debbie and me, as we realized that ultimately clinical management was not for us. I returned to being a full-time clinician, and Debbie took a role as lead nurse for clinical trials, leaving Elaine to run the unit with a new clinical director, David Howell. I felt a bit guilty for deserting her at the time, but I needn't have worried. Elaine, who'd already made an impact, never looked back. I have disagreed with her many times over the years and challenged her innovations, but to date she's never been wrong. To misquote Gore Vidal, 'when a colleague of mine succeeds a small part of me usually dies', but Elaine is one of the exceptions. I'll never tire of her winning awards and accolades; she deserves every one, and after all it was all down to me in the first place.

Elaine had already been planning for 'team and task' style working for the nurses at UCH since receiving guidance from the European Society of Intensive Care in the first week of March. She knew what had happened in Italy, she knew that there wouldn't be enough ICU nurses to continue one-to-one nursing and she knew that we'd have to adapt rapidly. There was no choice. She didn't want to change the way her staff worked, but she had to. It was either that or turn patients away at the front door, so for two weeks she'd been harassing her bosses for extra staff and resources and preparing her team. I was not surprised when they approached her to help head up nursing at the Nightingale.

'Wow, umm, so?' I replied, unhelpfully.

'I've got to give them an answer by lunchtime.'

'God. What do you want to do?'

'I don't want to go.'

Elaine had just returned from a six-month stint as interim head of nursing at the Lister Hospital, Stevenage. I'd been worried she'd not return from that; now she was being stolen again.

'Well, don't go, then.' I sounded like someone clinging to the threads of a dying relationship. 'I mean, you don't have to.'

'I know, but . . .'

'It's a huge honour?'

'I guess, and I don't know, maybe I should go. If they think . . . ?'

I got it. If they'd asked me to be clinical director of the Nightingale, I'd have felt conflicted. It was a massive project, a moment in history. It might be our generation's Dunkirk.

'You've got to do what you think's right. The unit would miss you, but . . . we'll be all right. We're used to you buggering off.'

'I wish they'd never asked.'

'Too good at your job.' I glanced at my watch. 'I've got to get to the SitRep meeting.'

'Oh, yeah, me too.'

'One thing I will say,' I added, working hard to avoid the tone of a spurned lover. 'It worries me, as a project.'

Later that day I passed her in the corridor, and with everything crossed behind my back, I raised an inquisitive eyebrow.

'I'm not going.'

'Thank fu— I mean, that's great. Great. God, that's a relief.'

The twice-daily Situation Report (SitRep) meetings were Rik's idea.

'OK,' he began, 'side room 1?'

I glanced at my handover sheet.

'Covid confirmed, ventilated.'

'Movable?'

'Ye . . . s.' I was struggling to read my own handwriting. 'Not peeing brilliantly.'

'We can filter in the Pods,' Steve (another ICU consultant) reminded me.

'OK, so yes, then.'

Steve put a purple V with an arrow next to it in the box marked SR 1 on the wall opposite.

We were in the ICU seminar room. One wall was plastered with white plastic sheets, on to which Rik had drawn a 6-foot-by-3-foot map of all the 100 potential ICU beds in the hospital.

Steve was Rik's right-hand man. While Rik is a ball of energy and invention, Steve is more considered, exploratory and lateral-thinking. An avid consumer of intellectual podcasts on his hour-long walk to work, he is modest, quietly spoken and never content with the status quo.

By the last week of March, the numbers of Covid patients at UCH was growing fast. Added to our baseline thirty-five beds within the four walls of the unit, we now had another forty-four ICU beds kitted out in the theatre complex (the Pods) and twenty CPAP beds up on the seventh floor.

The conversion of the seventh floor from a Hyper-Acute Stroke Unit (HASU) to a Covid CPAP unit was the brainchild of David.

To create the new unit David had first persuaded our sister hospital at Queen Square to temporarily house the HASU and then phoned Ronan Astin, a dynamic young respiratory physician, to see if he'd be happy to set up a CPAP unit in the soon-to-be-vacated space. Within a week (with the help of our ICU nurse consultant, John Welch) Ronan had converted the HASU into the High-Dependency Respiratory Unit (HDRU), and on 24 March the first patient came in through the door. No business case, no papers to the board, no arguments about budget lines, they just did it.

If Rik was leading us internally, David was looking at the bigger picture as our outward-facing boss. A week or so later he would take over as ICU lead for the whole of North Central London. Locally born and bred and UCH-trained, David knew the patch better than any of us, and he would use this, his boundless energy, considerable powers of persuasion and multiple phones to great effect over the next two months.

'Side room 2?' Rik asked.

'Query Covid, CPAP.'

'Ceilinged?'

'No . . . he's fifty-two.' My handwriting was getting more and more difficult to read, but my glasses just steamed up when I put them on over a mask.

Steve plucked an orange pen from his fist and wrote C in the box labelled SR 2.

'Duck?' Rik asked, tapping away at his laptop.

'Ducks' were patients with all the hallmarks of Covid who were yet to test positive – as per the old adage 'if it looks like a duck, and quacks like a duck – it's a duck'.

'Yes, still waiting for the first swab,' I looked down again at my sheet, 'but good story, and the chest x-ray's pretty convincing.'

'Lymphocytes?'

'Not sure, sorry. He only came in last night.'

'Low,' Tim confirmed via Zoom. 'And CRP's 230.'

'Thanks, Tim,' Rik called.

'So yeah, duck,' I confirmed.

'Mervyn?' It was Tim again. 'Can you move back? Sorry, all we can see at the moment is your belly.'

'Sorry, sorry.' Mervyn pushed his chair back away from the video camera.

'I'm trying to eat my breakfast.'

'Side room 3?' Rik ploughed on.

'Yup, non-Covid,' I confirmed, confidently. 'Pneumonia chap with C Diff, been here a month.'

'Might be going to the London Clinic,' David added via Zoom. Our nearest private ICU was now taking some of our non-Covid patients to help create capacity. 'Can you get another swab today? They need two negatives . . .'

'Sure. Great.'

The twice-daily SitRep meetings were now the cornerstones of our working day. Marshalled by Rik or Steve, the consultant in charge of each different area ran through the key details of every patient sequentially, while someone updated the wall plan with various symbols in a variety colours. Purple was confirmed Covid, blue confirmed non-Covid (rarely used by now) and orange, query Covid. The letter we used denoted the patient's ventilatory status (V - ventilated, C - CPAP, T – tracheostomy, etc.). Over time, we added annotations - 'RRT' for renal replacement therapy (the filter), an arrow for a potential bed move, a cap over the letter for patients with treatment limitations (ceilings) and so on.

The most challenging group were the query Covids. These were patients who had suspected Covid but were still awaiting a positive swab or, quite often, had tested negative. We could cohort confirmed Covid patients together in bays and likewise non-Covids, but we couldn't put query Covids in with either. They might be negative, so at risk of catching it, or positive and potential super-spreaders. They should, ideally be isolated in single rooms, but we only had eleven side rooms and they were labour-intensive to run. In an open bay experienced ICU nurses can be administering to one patient while keeping half an eye and ear on the patient next door, sometimes even on both sides. A solid wall between patients, however, makes it more difficult.

By now we'd unofficially divided the query Covids into 'possibles' and 'ducks'. The 'possibles' had enough features of Covid (perhaps a temperature and some respiratory symptoms) to warrant a test, but not the classic package. Over time they'd occasionally surprise us, so we had to take them seriously, but the emphasis was on protecting them from getting infected. The 'ducks', on the other hand, had classic Covid. The combination of a typical story, shadowing on chest x-ray and the right blood results meant Covid as far as we were concerned, but some of them tested negative, repeatedly, on throat swab. Most, eventually turned out to be positive, but the problem was where to put them in the meantime. In the end, with no other options, we created a bay for them: the 'Duck Pond'. It was imperfect, but pragmatic and unavoidable. To my knowledge no one ever caught Covid in the 'Duck Pond'.

With the wall map updated, the bed moves could be planned. By now the ICU itself was full, and each day we transferred ventilated patients across to the Pods and patients on CPAP upstairs to the HDRU. The priority was to free up side rooms for the next batch of ducks and possibles, but the challenge was finding appropriate people to move. The last thing a CPAP patient needed was to move out of ICU only to have to come back a day later to be intubated. Added to that, patients needed side rooms for other reasons. Some were immuno-compromised and some had infectious diarrhoea. In normal times all these patients would be in single rooms, but we only had what we had. Everything was a compromise.

After the SitRep meeting, I nipped back to the office to drop off my bag and bumped into Jamie, who was making a coffee in the galley kitchen off the main corridor.

'All right?' I asked,

'I'm below average. What do you think I should do?'

'Erm . . . ?'

'With people who asked to join one family but have now decided they'd rather be in a different one?'

'Sammy and Vuppe not getting on?'

'Hilarious. Although Sammy is a bit cross that Vuppe's got more Instagram followers.'

'Who wants to change team – sorry, *family*?'

'Thank you.' Jamie paused, 'Oh, you know, some people are struggling with resident nights. They think they'd be happier with the Westmoreland family.'

'You can choose your friends . . .'

'Is that meant to be helpful?'

'Sorry. Are the Westmoreland lot having the easiest time?'

'We've sent the oldies there, because there's no Covid.'

'That sounds fair enough.'

'They're doing shedloads of work. All the urgent cancer work. It's relentless.'

'Why don't you write one of your slightly sarcastic, passive-aggressive group emails?'

'Because I'm all about compassion now.' Jamie paused. 'I actually think people are being amazing. It's grim.'

'I know.'

As I donned to start my ward round that morning I couldn't get my conversation with Elaine and the whole Nightingale project out of my head. We'd seen a lot of patients by this time, and the more I saw the less convinced I was about the whole idea.

The first two patients I saw that day were both on CPAP. Fadi was a forty-four-year-old man of Lebanese heritage with a young daughter. (Another worry was the over-representation of non-Caucasians in our Covid ICU admissions. We didn't know why, but it was already clear that we were seeing far more people from ethnic minorities than we should have been – yet another confusing and alarming early feature of the pandemic.)

Fadi had had to close his café/restaurant when he'd fallen sick with Covid at the beginning of March but had assumed he'd just shake it off like most other people of his age and get back to work. He wasn't obese, or diabetic, or asthmatic, he was just non-Caucasian and unlucky. When I met him he'd been on CPAP for twenty-four hours and was holding his own physiologically, but he was terrified. At night, particularly, he became anxious, then agitated, and his breathing rate increased. For two days we calmed him down. We reassured him, gave him small doses of sedation, and he settled, but on the third day he started to tire, so I raised the possibility of putting him to sleep and taking over his breathing.

'Yes . . . please,' he replied.

As so often through the pandemic, I wasn't sure if it was the right thing at the right time, but he persuaded me. A couple of days later we transferred him over to the ICU in our sister hospital at Queen Square, which, along with the Pods, had become our overspill unit. I had a bad feeling as they wheeled him out the door. Adam was still fresh in my mind, and here was another one: young, fit and quickly on to a ventilator.

Opposite Fadi was Thanasis, a fifty-year-old man from Greece. Thanasis was a big man, over 6 feet tall and 16 stones, with jet-black hair. He'd moved with his wife to the UK three years before, got out of the restaurant business and set up his own transport company, but he still sang and played his bouzouki around the Greek eateries of North London. Previously he'd been fit and well, and for a couple of days he'd coped on CPAP, but then he too started to look tired. When I got to him that day he seemed to be dragging each breath into his lungs with his shoulders. He was sweaty, his oxygen requirements were increasing, and he'd had enough. He needed to be ventilated. I explained the situation to him, called the intubation team and left the bay to continue my ward round. An hour later I was called back, urgently.

In many ways Paavan is the quintessential anaesthetist. Smart, uncomplaining, unflustered and professional. When I walked back into the bay that day, he was ashen. I glanced around the bed. The two staff nurses and anaesthetic registrar looked equally traumatized.

'Hi. So?'

'The tube's in,' Paavan replied, 'it was difficult, but it's definitely in.' There was defiance in his voice.

I glanced up at the monitor and saw the turrets of carbon dioxide moving slowly across the screen. We measure carbon dioxide in the exhaled gas of each breath. It is the definitive test that your breathing tube is sitting in the trachea not the oesophagus, because the lungs produce carbon dioxide, whereas the stomach does not.

'But I can't get the sats up.'

My eyes moved up to the oxygen saturation – 75 per cent.

Normally, oxygen passes from the lungs into the blood, where it binds to the molecule haemoglobin. The haemoglobin then transports the oxygen to the tissues. The saturation monitor (the clothes peg with the red light that they put on your finger when they check your 'Obs' or 'Vitals' as the Americans say) measures the percentage of haemoglobin that is carrying or 'saturated' with oxygen. The normal figure is 96–99 per cent. When the oxygen saturation drops, the note of the monitor's 'beep' drops too, from a crisp, reassuring, high-pitched 'ting' all the way down to a miserable dirge-like tone, not dissimilar to the beginning of the death march from *Star Wars*. A drop in oxygen saturation during an intubation is not uncommon. Often there is a period of no ventilation as the tube is manoeuvred into the trachea, but below 90 per cent the rate of fall accelerates, and the anaesthetist starts to sweat. Through our training we become hard-wired to the note of that 'beep.' Below 50 per cent, the heart slows, and the true character of the anaesthetist is revealed. Once the tube is in, however, and the lungs are ventilated again, the oxygen levels usually pick up very quickly. Not with Thanasis. The tube was definitely in, and he was being ventilated with 100 per cent oxygen, but his blood oxygen levels were not budging.

As I would later find out, Paavan and the team had just been through twenty-five minutes of misery. While they'd still been assembling their equipment and going through the checklist, Thanasis's oxygen levels had dropped, so they'd been rushed. They'd then followed standard procedure, but despite that, once asleep, Thanasis's oxygen levels plummeted further, and the first attempt to place the tracheal tube failed. They used a bag and facemask to ventilate while preparing for a second attempt and were partially successful, but still the oxygen levels remained perilously low, around 60 per cent. A second failed attempt at intubation was followed by insertion of a laryngeal mask (an airway device that sits at the back of the throat), but still the oxygen saturations would not rise. Finally, having called for more equipment, they got a tube in. It must have felt like the longest twenty-five minutes of their lives.

We talk about human factors, crisis management and controlled and uncontrolled situations. They'd never worked together, so they had never had the chance to build up trust and understanding. They weren't even sure of each other's job titles and they were in full PPE, struggling right on the edge of control for every one of those twenty-five minutes.

When I am in those situations, there's usually a moment when I question myself.

'How did I get to this point? What did I do wrong? What if he dies? Have I been negligent? How negligent? What will I say to his family? How will they react? Will they believe we really did everything possible? Will my colleagues stand up for me in court? What do they actually think of me? Do I have a good reputation? Would I survive in prison?'

It's uncomfortable to admit this. Obviously I'm not proud of it, but I don't think it's unusual for ICU doctors to think this way. I do worry deeply about the fate of the person in front of me, independent of its impact on my life, but it is confusing, because in that moment our fates are so entangled. The fear and dread is for the patient mainly, but also a bit for me. Maybe more than a bit. When you witness a stranger's tragedy and the emotion is sadness, it's simple, but if you play an active part in that tragedy, the emotions are much more complex, however good your intentions. When I hear about a friend who has had a patient do badly, my concern is not just for the patient, it is also for the friend. How are they? I know it is worse for the patient, obviously, but I also know that my friend will have been doing their best. We are all acutely aware that something could go wrong for any of us at any time. When it happens to a friend we are reminded of our vulnerability. We can immediately imagine what they are feeling.

However, I don't think that the invasion of these selfish thoughts is detrimental to the care we deliver. If anything, it focuses the mind. There's no conflict of interests, our goals and the patient's are completely aligned, our fate relies on theirs. That is, until the fear and anxiety get out of control and we freeze in the moment or longer term, start to avoid risky situations, challenging cases and difficult decisions – 'lose our nerve'. Then, there is a problem, and that is why Paavan and all like him – the people who step forward when it gets tough – must be treasured.

But this wasn't my mess, it was someone else's. I'm not saying Paavan had caused a mess, he absolutely had not. He'd got the tube in, and the patient was still alive, but joining when I did, I was taking up the knight in shining armour role. Clear-headed, fresh, guilt-free, I could only make things better – or so I thought.

'Tube's definitely not in too far?' I asked,

'Twenty-three centimetres at the lips, both sides of the chest are moving,' Paavan replied.

It is easy to push the endo-tracheal tube in too far, especially when it has been difficult to site. The tip then slips beyond the trachea and down into the right lung, meaning that the left lung receives no ventilation. Pull it back a couple of centimetres and things dramatically improve. Paavan had already thought of that. The tube was not in too far.

'Fully paralysed?'

'Yup.'

'Tried a recruitment manoeuvre?'

'Yeah, he hated it.'

Putting higher pressure into the lungs for a minute or two sometimes 'recruits' or expands up collapsed air spaces and improves the transfer of oxygen into the circulation. On the other hand, it can just cause the blood pressure to collapse. It had not worked for Thanasis.

'Chest x-ray?'

'I've called for one.'

'I don't think it's going to change anything right now,' I mumbled, going through an algorithm of options in my head. 'His chest's moving fine.'

'But the sats are still 75,' the bedside staff nurse countered.

A chest x-ray might reveal something unexpected, air escaped around the lung or a blocked-off airway, but I didn't think so in this case, and we needed to do something now. I was quickly running out of ideas.

'There's nothing to suction? Thick secretions?'

'Hardly anything.'

'OK.' I looked briefly around my colleagues. 'We're going to have to turn him over, now. Have we got enough people?'

Turning people on to their front, or 'proning' them, often improves the oxygen levels dramatically. Within five minutes, Paavan had secured the tracheal tube, we'd put protection over the eyes, pillows on to his chest and pelvis, sorted out his lines, infusions and catheter and assembled seven of us around the bed space. Thanasis was 16 stones. We went through the checklist, wrapped him in two sheets, twisted the edges together to make a 'Cornish pasty,' slid him to the edge of the bed, turned him to 90 degrees, checked all the lines and tubes again and then pulled him through on to his front. I glanced at the carbon dioxide trace to check we were still ventilating him, then looked up at the oxygen saturation and waited.

74 per cent . . . 73 per cent . . . 71 per cent . . .

'Can you try it on a different finger?'

Sometimes if the blood flow to a particular finger is poor, the oxygen saturation reads artificially low. After a few seconds it picked up the trace on a second finger.

69 per cent . . . 67 per cent . . .

'We'll give it a minute. Maybe it was just the turning itself.'

65 per cent . . . 63 per cent . . .

I looked up at Paavan. This was very much my mess now, not his.

'Could the tube have moved?' I asked.

Paavan looked down at the breathing tube he was still clutching between his fingers.

'Still 23 at the lips, and the chest's moving nicely.'

'Sats are 60 per cent.'

'Shit, right.' I took another deep breath. 'OK, we'll have to turn him back over. Can someone ask for the nitric?'

Inhaled nitric oxide crosses from the air spaces to the blood vessels in the lungs and dilates them, thus increasing the flow of blood and often improving blood oxygen levels. It has never been shown to save lives, but at that moment I didn't care. I was willing to try anything.

By the time we turned Thanasis face up again his lips were slate-grey, but gradually his oxygen levels did start to increase. Four of us stared at the monitor, willing them to go on climbing, and over the next twenty minutes they inched up to 78 per cent – still frighteningly low, but moving in the right direction. Then, with the help of nitric oxide, they climbed further, up to the mid 80s. It was time to stop fiddling. He was safe – for now.

As Paavan and I pulled off our PPE, neither of us thought Thanasis would survive. Almost worse was the fear he'd survive but be left brain damaged. He'd been more than an hour with dangerously low oxygen levels. The effect of that on the brain is unpredictable – some people come through unscathed, but many don't.

'Well done,' I mumbled. 'Are you . . . ?'

'Going to intubate the lady in bay 3?' Paavan replied. 'Yeah, I just need a quick drink.'

'Thanks. Have you got a team? Do you want me to . . . ?'

'No, no we'll be fine.'

A slug of water, and Paavan was off to put a breathing tube into the next profoundly hypoxic patient, while I went to continue my ward round.

Whenever I see Paavan now, in the corridor or the coffee room, those forty-five minutes with Thanasis flash through my mind. His too, perhaps. The team of intubators at UCH were universally fantastic, the epitome of calm under pressure. They never missed a tube. Every patient was successfully intubated and stabilized, despite many intubations being as terrifying as Thanasis's.

The problem was that I couldn't see how Thanasis or Fadi or John or any of the other patients we had on the ICU at the time could be managed at the Nightingale. They wouldn't have fitted the criteria. They were either on CPAP, which the Nightingale did not offer, or too sick and unstable to be looked after safely with the facilities and model of care they proposed.

As I heard and read more about the project through the last week of March, I became increasingly concerned. Not only was I worried about patients going to the Nightingale, I was also worried about the effect it would have on our own hospital. The trained staff for this new venture had to come from somewhere, and the plan was that they would come out of the ICUs around London. As the Nightingale filled up, our staff would be redeployed. We weren't quite sure how this would happen, but as we understood it, there wouldn't be a choice. A certain number of staff would have to go. Like it or not, we'd be managing more and more patients with less and less staff, and they'd need equipment too. The impact on our hospital, physically and psychologically, would be immense.

The logic was that there should be parity of care across all ICUs. If the Nightingale was running on one trained nurse to six patients and one consultant to forty-two patients, then all the other hospitals should be prepared to do the same. Staff must be spread thinly everywhere. I understood the ethical premise – everyone should receive equal care – and I understood the motive – no one who might benefit should be denied ICU support – but for me there was a third factor to consider. What if you couldn't look after critically ill Covid ICU patients in this way? What if they were just too sick, too unstable and too unpredictable? What if offering thousands of them 'ICU-lite' meant that a high proportion died? What if, by taking staff out of hospitals to work at the Nightingale, you actually did more harm than good?

I have great respect for the people behind the Nightingale project. Some I know personally, some by reputation. They are eminent, distinguished, clever people, and what they achieved in two weeks was extraordinary. The potential scale of the crisis was unimaginable, and their speed of thought and action remarkable, but by the end of March I felt that our understanding of the disease had changed. It wasn't a single-organ lung disease. It caused a spectrum of problems, from people who needed just oxygen or CPAP to those profoundly sick and unstable, often in multiple organ failure. The Nightingale group in the middle, who just needed some time on a simple anaesthetic machine ventilator, didn't really seem to exist. As more and more patients came in through the door, this group still failed to materialize.

I wasn't suggesting that we shouldn't create extra capacity, I was just proposing a different model, or at the very least a modification of their model. My preference was that we should expand the ICUs in base hospitals as much as we possibly could and then, when absolutely necessary, use the Nightingale as a 'Covid field hospital'. A proportion of patients with a good story for Covid ('ducks'), who were not *in extremis*, would be taken straight there by paramedics. If this was logistically too difficult, they could go via Emergency Departments, but, either way, transfer to the Nightingale would be early, when the patients were awake and breathing for themselves, as opposed to when they were already sedated and ventilated. A triage team would then greet them and divide them into groups. Those who needed just oxygen would be housed in a 'ward' area, those who required CPAP, in a smaller high-dependency unit (HDU) and those who went on to need intubation and ventilation in an even smaller ICU. From what we knew already, the split should be roughly 70 per cent ward: 15 per cent HDU and 15 per cent ICU. The patients who required just oxygen would benefit as they could receive oxygen safely with low staffing ratios. Those who required CPAP could also be managed safely and still use relatively low nurse-to-patient ratios, perhaps 1:6. There is precedent for this, and crucially the use of CPAP would reduce the number who required full ventilation, but those who did could then receive the highest concentration of resources available. The base hospitals around London would then focus on expanding their ICU capacity to take as many of the sickest and most complex patients as possible, some of whom might be transfers back from the Nightingale. This model had many problems, but it felt to me like the least bad option.

By the time we had significant numbers of ICU patients at the Nightingale, there would have been rationing. Vital equipment would have run out, and the government knew this, so they put out a call for companies to make ventilators.

'You make them, we'll buy them,' Matt Hancock proclaimed,

but what he didn't know at the time was that the ventilators for Covid patients needed to be highly sophisticated, proper ICU ventilators. Added to that, there would not have been enough kidney machines, syringe drivers or trained ICU nurses. The more people you ventilated, the more of all these you needed (to keep them asleep, manage their other organs and look after them).

Even at the surge intensity we reached there were shortages. Ramani Moonesinghe and the team at NHS England did an amazing job of distributing equipment as widely and equitably as they could every day, but there was only so much they could do. The whole world wanted ICU ventilators. I was convinced CPAP had a place in the management of Covid, it seemed to be good for many patients and to preserve ventilators, but the Nightingale model was encouraging people to bypass CPAP and put patients straight on to the ventilator. If your hospital was overwhelmed and the only overflow facility required patients to be intubated and ventilated, then that's what you'd do.

For me we were better to let the base hospitals do as much of the ICU as possible; to keep their teams together in a familiar environment; to redeploy staff within the hospital, staff already familiar with the computer systems, the labs and radiology; to keep people with the leaders and managers they knew and trusted; to keep the sickest people in institutions with other specialists – anaesthetists, surgeons, cardiologists, haematologists and chest physicians; to let an already established system of ICU expand.

On Friday, 27 March Boris Johnson tested positive for Covid, and Chief Medical Officer Chris Whitty went into self-isolation. By now 759 people had died with Covid in the UK, 180 in London alone. The pandemic was rapidly gaining momentum. London Mayor Sadiq Khan warned us to expect 'a large number of deaths' and the Nightingale was being talked of as the solution to all our problems. That morning Professor Monty Mythen called me. Monty, a colleague and mentor over the years, had been asked to join the Care Quality Commission's (CQC) visit to the Nightingale the following Tuesday. He'd caught Covid early and was still quite ill so, knowing that I was interested in the subject, suggested I take his place.

I looked around the sea of faces. We'd come back up from the huge 'Barn ICU' to the Nightingale's operation hub. A couple of years earlier I'd sat in this very room, listening to a lecture about the latest experimental ICU treatment to fail. Teams of people were working in huddles around tables. These were the key players, each grappling with different aspects of the monumental challenge they all faced. In five days' time they'd be open, admitting their first patient. I spotted a pharmacist from UCH and nodded. Builders, soldiers, nurses, management consultants, security guards, paramedics, executives, doctors, physiotherapists and a myriad of others criss-crossed the room, energized and focused. The 'can do' attitude was tangible.

'So please, ask questions. Talk to whomever you'd like,' our host offered, his arms spread wide.

'Could I speak to the intensivists, if they've got time?' I asked, tentatively.

'Sure, over there, go for it.'

I made my way over to the two consultant intensivists in the far corner of the room and over the next forty-five minutes outlined my well-rehearsed arguments. They were patient, accommodating, engaged and thoughtful, but they didn't agree.

At 4 p.m., the CQC team huddled around a table to discuss our findings. I was the only intensivist, but the experience in the room was impressive. These people knew how to assess a hospital and cut quickly to the chase. I listened, feeling very much the junior partner until eventually they asked me what I thought. So I told them.

That night I didn't sleep well. Was I right? Was the Nightingale really such a disaster, or was I just being a pain in the arse? Maybe, but I couldn't get away from the fact that it felt like a huge risk, so I called Professor Geoff Bellingan. Geoff is another ICU colleague, but more importantly medical director at UCH and well known around London. People would listen to him. He was still recuperating from a knee replacement, but luckily he's a workaholic and was already re-engaged in non-clinical work. He asked typically incisive questions, mulled it over and then promised he'd go away and talk to people. He had access to people, important people. If anyone could influence this, he could.

I wasn't privy to discussions after that and I don't claim that my nagging altered anything, but I do know that there was a change of strategy. Hospitals did not want to give up their staff and equipment, and consensus was reached around London that we should try as far as possible to keep the ICU patients within established hospitals. The Nightingale model did not change, but the surge and super-surge capacity of each hospital was re-evaluated, smaller hospitals were supported by their bigger local teaching hospitals, and specialist transfer teams moved carefully selected patients to units with the appropriate facilities. UCH, being big and new, had relatively greater ability to expand, and over the next three weeks, marshalled by David, we accepted forty-seven patients from other hospitals. Our sister hospital at Queen Square took another twenty. North Central London sector transferred eighty-seven patients in total, twelve to the Nightingale. Assuming the four other sectors transferred similar numbers, that's roughly 400 transfers around London. The Nightingale admitted just over fifty.

My feelings about the Nightingale have changed over the

months. I don't have remorse about voicing my concerns, and I am glad that we managed to keep most ICU patients within established hospitals, but so are the people who built it. As they said when we visited: 'The best outcome would be if this ends up a big white elephant. We'd be delighted.'

I am grateful that there was a back-up hospital, just in case the worst predictions were realized and I don't know which model would have worked best, but my overwhelming emotion, looking back, is relief that we didn't end up needing 4,000 extra ICU beds during the first surge.

I remember sitting in our chief executive's office a day or two after my Nightingale visit with Rik, David and the clinical director of the Emergency Department. The subject under discussion was super-surge: how many ICU beds could we surge to if the shit hit the fan – really hit it. If lockdown made no difference to the doubling rate. Looking out of the window at the deserted streets, it seemed impossible that lockdown would not have an impact, but we had no idea how much, so it had to be modelled. Rik and Marcel Levi, the chief executive, had come up with a figure of 250 ICU beds for UCH. Our ICU has thirty-five beds and is already considered large; most district general hospitals have about twelve. 250 ICU patients in one building was unimaginable, but Marcel, Rik and David were deadly serious. If we were going to avoid using the Nightingale, this was what we must prepare for.

4. Decisions

2 April 2020

'I'm going to move on from rotas, if that's OK – to the clinical . . .'

'Just one more thing.' Alice smiled, apologetically, 'before we leave rotas.' She paused. 'Some of the anaesthetists are struggling.'

It was 5.10 on 2 April 2020; another ICU consultants meeting. I'd been chairing two of these a week for the last three weeks. I'm not the leader, not even a leader, but I can chair a meeting. I have a talent for it. I was told so on a leadership course in 2009. It's not the talent I'd have chosen – I'd have taken Peter Cook's or Roger Federer's – but I have what I have, and back then there were a lot of meetings to be chaired.

By now 600 people a day were dying with Covid in the UK. Matt Hancock, the health secretary, had just returned to work after his brush with the virus and quickly announced a target of 25,000 tests per day by the end of the month. He also wrote off £13.4 billion of NHS debt as both British Airways and Nissan announced plans to furlough thousands of staff.

I was keen to move on to the clinical issues and determined to finish by six, but I couldn't ignore the anaesthetists.

'Because . . . ?' I asked.

'They're doing more resident nights than us, and some feel patronized, some want more support.'

People started to chip in from around the room.

'So we need to support some of them more and some of them . . . less?'

'They feel some of us are more supportive than others.'

'So some of us need to support some of them more, but . . .'

I understood why the anaesthetists were unhappy. I'd spoken to them and I am one. They may have all worked in intensive care during their training, but as consultants they'd chosen not to.

It's Marmite, ICU – you either love it or you don't. Most anaesthetists don't and choose to subspecialize in something else such as pain medicine or paediatrics. Working on a ward where the mortality is 20 per cent, in normal times, and probably nearer 40 per cent for Covid patients, isn't everyone's cup of tea, but suddenly fifty anaesthetists had become full-time intensivists. Over half of those were consultants, many in their forties and fifties. Some had not worked in ICU for twenty years. The majority were working in the Pods, a stuffy, windowless space, designed to accommodate people after their hip replacements for some painkillers and a cup of tea on their way back to the ward.

Over the next two weeks the number of Pod patients would swell to twenty-seven, some in what was paediatric recovery, some in operating theatres, some in a pre-operative holding bay. None of these areas had windows, but all had been converted into pop-up ICUs. A combination of PPE and geography made communication with the outside world almost impossible – communicating with someone standing next to you was hard enough. The anaesthetists were on gruelling thirteen-hour shifts, every fifth night it was a night shift. They were working with nurses they'd never met, and the equipment changed every day as we begged and borrowed more ventilators, infusion pumps and dialysis machines from GOSH, the Royal National Orthopaedic Hospital, the local private hospitals, even China, Japan and Germany. They were being ordered around by colleagues who were often twenty years their junior and had little more understanding of how to manage this terrible new disease than they did, because none of us knew how to manage it, it was new. I understood why they were not happy, but I didn't have the solution.

'They wrote their own rotas, didn't they?' a voice asked over Zoom.

'Sort of . . .' I began.

'. . . and *we* need to be here more in the daytime. We're in different roles.'

These arguments would go round and round throughout the surge of Covid cases in early April. Every staff group had a different set of pressures, and within each group there were as many opinions as there were people. Everyone was willing, but also stressed, scared and out of their depth, and with more than forty consultants working on ICU now (up from our usual eighteen), consensus was often impossible. By solving one person's problem you inevitably upset someone else. It was whack-a-mole.

'OK,' I sighed, 'I'll talk to James and Viki, find out more, but in the meantime can we all just try to be as flexible and understanding as possible?'

'I do think it's important that we're in charge.'

I bit my tongue. It was a fair point, in a way. The buck did stop with us, the regular intensivists. It was our responsibility to oversee the management plans and to make the strategic decisions, but we were working in a new world and we had to work as a team, as equals. We were completely reliant on their experience, their counsel, their ability to look after unstable physiology and to deal with life-threatening emergencies, their knowledge and their wisdom. While the intensivists rotated through different sections of the ICU, the anaesthetists were working full-time in the Pods. They knew these cases intimately. They'd got used to each patient's quirks and fluctuations. And there were far too many patients for us to manage on our own. This was not the time to fall out.

'Remember they're very experienced anaesthetists, many of them, and they've gone back to a job they actively chose not to do.' I didn't leave time for a reply. 'Now, I want to move on to the clinical. CPAP.'

There were nine of us in the room and another five connecting remotely on Zoom. The other four consultants who should have been in attendance were off with Covid – one significantly ill. We did our best to social distance from each other, but I think we felt that we needed to be there. Some people joined meetings by Zoom, and we wiped surfaces and our phones, bags and wallets, but few wore masks outside of patient areas (the prevailing view at the time was that they made little difference), and regularly there were eight or nine of us in our office.

Some people were fatalistic. They'd become resigned to the fact that we were all bound to get Covid at some point, so why fight it? In the end eight out of the eighteen of us tested positive for Covid in the first surge, although most probably caught it outside of work.

By now we had all become full-time intensivists; from the sixty-two-year-old professor (who was determined to do his bit, despite our protestations) to the brand-new locum, on a full shift pattern. Between shifts we each worked on different aspects of the Covid response, but everything else had been dropped; research, education, anaesthesia, clinics, audit, quality improvement – there was only Covid now.

As intensivists we are used to sick patients, but normally we share their care with the primary team; leukaemics with the haematologist, patients with pancreatitis with the gastro-enterologist, etc. With Covid it was different. We were the primary team. They were cared for by the physicians when they were on the normal ward, but the only effective therapy at the time was oxygen, and when that was not enough they came to ICU.

It is a privilege to work alongside all the world-class experts in their respective fields at UCH, but none of them could really help us now. They had ideas and theories about what might help, but no evidence to back them up. Covid was the only thing that anyone was talking about, anywhere, and it was ours. We had the biggest cohort of the sickest patients we'd ever seen and we were desperately trying to work out how to manage them. Today the question was CPAP.

'Three things we need to discuss,' I continued. 'Firstly, are we doing the right thing? I mean is it actually good for patients to keep them awake on CPAP? Secondly, have we got the oxygen supply to continue with this strategy? And thirdly, do we want to join a trial comparing it with early intubation?'

CPAP (the 'head out of the car window on the motorway therapy') is an established treatment for sleep apnoea and heart failure. It is also often used to open up the collapsed lung bases of patients after major surgery. The idea of treating Covid with CPAP was that it would open up airspaces that have collapsed due to inflammation and secretions and so allow more oxygen to be transferred into the bloodstream. It might also reduce the work of breathing and make patients less breathless. However, at the beginning of the outbreak the national advice was to avoid it.

The logic for avoiding it was that it would only delay the inevitable. If the patient needed CPAP, sooner or later they'd need intubation, so why wait until they were even sicker, and the intubation even higher risk? I had sympathy with this argument – we'd had some hairy intubations, Thanasis a case in point – but that wasn't the only concern. Allowing people to go on breathing for themselves on CPAP might increase the pressures across the lung tissues and perpetuate the inflammation, whereas putting patients to sleep and gently ventilating the lungs, might minimize the inflammation and optimize the chance of recovery. There was also the theoretical risk to staff. CPAP masks leak, and the high gas flow they require might propel the virus into the environment, whereas intubated patients are ventilated via a sealed system of tubing, so the virus should be contained. The final consideration was oxygen. Most CPAP devices require high-flow oxygen to function, particularly to deliver the high settings required for Covid. Some machines need more than 100 litres of oxygen per minute. If you suddenly fired up thirty more of those on a ward, you could quickly drain a hospital's oxygen supply, and that would be catastrophic.

Most of the UK accepted this advice, but Professor Mervyn Singer at UCH, who had been speaking to twelve of his professorial friends in Italy, had other ideas. Italy was three weeks ahead of us and already at peak surge when he'd spoken to them in mid March. They had vital experience and they'd told him to go for CPAP. In their units, the use of CPAP avoided the need for intubation in about half the patients. For that 50 per cent, the positive pressure via a mask or hood was enough. They argued that this was not only good for those patients, but also preserved their most precious resource – ICU ventilators. They'd also reassured him that their staff were not catching Covid from patients (so far). Their ICU beds were not filled with ICU doctors and nurses.

We were convinced by this story and, being a big new hospital, we had good oxygen supplies, so we'd gone down the CPAP route. Our unit was an outlier in the UK, but we'd seen successes. The first few patients we put on CPAP had done well. They avoided being put on a ventilator, got better and went home; John was a good example. I was convinced (and it was part of the reason I'd been so worried about the Nightingale) but then I'd looked after Fadi and Thanasis. They'd tolerated CPAP initially and stabilized, but were both now on ventilators. Had we done them a disservice? Would they have been better served by being intubated earlier? Did the benefit of CPAP to some outweigh the possible harm to others? Nobody knew.

We claim to practise evidence-based medicine, to seek out the best evidence, assess it objectively and modify our practice accordingly. The truth is we interpret the evidence to fit our own experience, beliefs and biases. Until the evidence is overwhelming we stick to what we think we know, and in ICU there is so little evidence that is overwhelming. In Covid ICU there was none. We tried to extrapolate from our understanding of other diseases and from plausible biological theories, but it soon became apparent that this disease was different. It was so unpredictable, severe, prolonged, fluctuant and just odd.

Happy hypoxia made no sense. Why did patients with catastrophically low oxygen levels, who should have been gasping for air, turn up reporting only mild breathlessness? Why did patients on maximal CPAP and breathing frighteningly fast happily text their friends and give the thumbs-up when they should have been exhausted and begging to be put to sleep? Should we treat the patient or the numbers? If the patient felt fine, were they? Or did the numbers know better? We didn't know. Sometimes they were fine, sometimes they weren't.

At UCH we'd decided to treat the patient. We were giving CPAP and accepting this strange new world that we didn't really understand, as long as the patient was giving us the 'thumbs up'. We were acutely aware, however, that south of the river at St Thomas's, if you required more than 40 per cent oxygen via a normal facemask, you were put to sleep, intubated and ventilated. They'd seen more Covid patients than us and they were convinced that their strategy worked. It was too early for any meaningful comparisons in outcomes.

There were also logistical considerations. Many smaller hospitals in London had already run out of capacity. The early intubation strategy meant they'd filled their ICUs with sedated, ventilated patients very quickly, and still the patients kept coming. They'd put the next wave into operating theatres on anaesthetic machines, but even those spaces were now full. They couldn't take any more. They'd run out of kit, space and staff – within days.

An ICU ventilator is a complex piece of equipment. The settings can be manipulated to match precisely the requirement of an individual patient. They are designed to ventilate people with severely damaged lungs for weeks, months even. Anaesthetic machines, on the other hand, have relatively simple ventilators designed to push oxygen, air and anaesthetic gases into patients with normal lungs for a few hours. Covid patients were being ventilated on anaesthetic machines because that was all hospitals had left, but it had already become apparent that for many Covid cases they were just not up to the job.

The size of UCH, combined with our preparation and CPAP policy, meant that, relatively speaking, we had retained capacity. We'd managed to maintain the flow of patients through the main ICU and out into the Pods and HDRU, always having just about enough equipment and staff. We were stretched. Our nursing ratios had dipped to one ICU nurse per four patients, but we were still in a better position than a lot of hospitals in North London. As a result, we could pursue our strategy of trying to keep the sickest patients within established hospitals by transferring many into UCH. If we'd intubated early this would not have been possible (although in different circumstances St Thomas' Hospital also accepted many transfers), but did that justify potential harm to some individual patients?

We're a cohesive group, the UCH ICU consultants. There are strong personalities, gripes and certainly no shortage of opinions, but we respect and like each other. It's an impressive bunch of people: four professors, a rising star of education, a shining light in clinical trials, some leading data scientists, an IT genius, a couple of international names in peri-operative medicine and a world-class meetings-chairperson. More importantly they are all clinicians I'd happily let take care of me, and the pandemic had galvanized us. The office was buzzing, we were getting through coffee pods like never before (another of my responsibilities) and we had been enacting decisions at a speed we'd previously only dreamed of, but the optimal clinical management of Covid was a matter of opinion, and in this group there was inevitably a range of opinions.

A small team of three were almost constantly reviewing the medical journals and national guidance, trying to come up with evidence-based recommendations, but as yet there was no real evidence, and as, individually, we acquired more anecdotal experience of this baffling, energy-sapping disease, it became increasingly challenging to agree. We were each scarred by different experiences.

'Yes, we are doing the right thing, yes, there is enough oxygen, and no to the trial,' Rik proposed.

They were off. Time to up my chairing skills a notch.

'Thanks, Rik. OK, can we have David, then Mervyn, then Sam?'

'It's completely saving the sector . . .'

'There is no evidence it causes harm.'

A classic use of the lack of evidence to push one's own evidence-free argument.

'From the echoes I've done so far . . .'

Sam could bring almost any conversation back to his favourite topic, echocardiography – ultrasound scans of the heart.

'Thanks, Sam. Steve?'

'The truth is we don't know.'

A typical note of caution from Steve, but it was soon apparent that no one wanted to throw CPAP in the bin.

'So is oxygen consumption OK with our use of CPAP?' I asked.

'Not a problem. I'm monitoring it,' Rik confirmed.

'But the low-oxygen alarms were going off constantly in the Pods, overnight,' Sam countered.

'Ignore them.'

'Ignore them?' I queried. I trust Rik implicitly, but ignoring low-oxygen alarms went against everything I'd ever learned.

'It sounds worse than it . . .' Rik paused 'they're set to alarm at pretty high pressures, so as long as the ventilators are still working . . .'

The room fell uncharacteristically silent.

'It'll be fine.' Rik was ready to move on.

'OK, great.' I, on the other hand, wasn't quite ready. 'But just out of interest, what do we do if the ventilators do stop working. In the middle of the night, say?'

'Won't happen, call me. Oh, and when Mervyn's mark 2 gizmo comes out, the oxygen consumption will actually fall.'

'Mercedes say Monday,' Mervyn confirmed. He, Dave Brealey, UCL and the German car manufacturers had managed to transform an old, redundant piece of kit into an effective, mass-producible CPAP device – in a week. Mark 1 worked fine but required a high flow rate of oxygen. Mark 2 didn't even need very much oxygen. To date over 2,000 models have been distributed to 110 hospitals in the UK and the design circulated, free of charge, around the world.

'Good, so call Rik when the ventilators fail.' I was being facetious but I had complete faith. 'And finally, the trial?'

'Are you happy to intubate people who are sitting comfortably on 50 per cent oxygen?' Dave asked, typically cutting to the chase.

No one was, and so the CPAP discussion was done. I still felt slightly uneasy, but their arguments were sound, consensus was vital, and I was on schedule. And there was no evidence, of course, either way.

'Good so, next item – proning.'

Proning is an established ICU intervention. It is a surprise to many relatives, a shock to some, and one poor woman misheard and spent a terrible couple of days desperately trying to work out how and why we were 'pruning' her father.

There was already evidence for proning. It doesn't always work, as Thanasis dramatically demonstrated, but pre-Covid controlled trials in patients with severe lung injury revealed that it not only improves oxygen levels in most people, but also increases their chance of surviving. However, for years the ICU community has largely ignored this evidence because proning is labour-intensive and not without risk. The turn itself requires six people and scrupulous attention to detail, and then, when on their front, patients are more difficult to assess and thus more vulnerable. The eyes and face are at increased risk of pressure sores, and each two-hourly head turn requires an anaesthetist to manage the breathing tube. If that comes out, when the patient is face down it is likely to be fatal. In the last few years, however, the evidence had overwhelmed us, and we'd started to prone more and more. The word from Italy and China was that Covid patients responded particularly well. They liked to be on their front.

Proning works by improving the match of ventilation to blood flow in the lungs. Blood flows preferentially downhill, to the back of the lungs, but these areas are likely to be the most inflamed and collapsed, so the ventilation occurs mainly to the front. To get oxygen from the lungs to the circulation you need the blood flow and ventilation in the same place. When you turn people on to their front, for a while the worst inflammation is now at the top, so the blood flow and ventilation are matched at the bottom, and the oxygen levels in the blood rise. It is more complicated than that, but the key thing is that it makes sense and it works. The regime is twice-daily turns, sixteen hours on their front, eight hours on their back. In normal times we might have one or two people being proned at any one time on our ICU. With Covid we had up to twenty-five. In normal times the decision would be carefully thought through. With Covid we were having to turn people as emergencies, often in the middle of the night – a life-saving manoeuvre to get the oxygen levels up. We had teams of medical students and surgeons roaming the units twice a day just to turn people over.

'OK.' I had timetabled a maximum of fifteen minutes for proning. 'So the questions are, at what oxygen threshold? For how many days? Do we emergency late-prone? And do we prone with tracheys in? Yes, Dave.'

'Ten days and stop.'

'Sam, then Steve.'

'Even if they're still responding?'

'Do we continue proning for ten days, even if it doesn't seem to be helping?' Steve paused and scratched his head. I waited. 'Could it be helping in ways we can't see?'

I had no idea, so I moved on.

'Alice.'

'We've seen horrible pressure sores and eye damage, I think we keep it as simple as possible, seven days maximum and stop. If it's going to work it will have, there is no evidence beyond . . .'

And so it went on. There were no right or wrong answers, and as ever no evidence, but we had to do something. We found a compromise (within fifteen minutes – I thank you) and agreed an oxygen threshold, ten days as the standard course, but with flexibility depending on the situation. Like so much of the clinical management we were scrabbling around in the dark or, to put more optimistically, learning rapidly on the job. We parked the issue of proning people with tracheostomies because no one had had a tracheostomy yet, and we left the issue of emergency late-proning unresolved. It was something we'd all end up doing at some point over the next few weeks, when we'd run out of other ideas.

I liked Alice's concept of keeping it as simple as possible. It made sense. We should do simple things well, avoid harm, not get too fancy, keep it protocolized as much as possible and give the already stretched nurses a chance. The problem was that the disease was not simple. If you just did simple things, it seemed to laugh in your face. The patients were too sick, for too long, and too fragile and unpredictable. There wasn't a simple solution, as far as I could see, much as I'd have loved there to have been. This was a feature of Covid that we hadn't appreciated until we saw it up close and personal. It wasn't just the number of Covid patients that were coming to ICU, it was also how complex and gruelling so many of them were to manage. As Adam had demonstrated, it was affecting not just the lungs, but also the brain, the heart, the kidneys, the guts, everything. Just when you thought you'd got a plan and were winning, they'd do something totally unexpected and make you rethink everything. I could barely imagine what it was like for their families trying to make sense of it all back at home.

We went on to discuss one more clinical issue, the fact that Covid patients seemed to be particularly vulnerable to blood clots, and then moved on – ahead of time. I was on fire.

'Good. Clinical done, so now trainees and any urgent AOBs. I think we'll have to leave relatives, PPE and nurses until Thursday.'

These meetings had an unlimited scope: clinical management, rotas, redeployment, data, estates, research, equipment, transfers, relatives, staff wellbeing, staff testing, training, pathways, PPE, ethics, pay, IT . . . the list went on. In some ways it felt as if we were running the hospital.

'So, Alice, two minutes on trainees. Problems?'

'Thanks! Umm yes, nightmare.' Alice looked down at her spreadsheets, 'I mean not the trainees, they're great on the whole, but I've totally messed up their rota. The exams are all off, rotations are cancelled, leave's cancelled, interviews are generally on hold, and they're all wrestling with the whole Nightingale decision.'

'Have any gone to the Nightingale?'

'Not yet, but some have asked me.'

'Nooo!'

'I said you'd be there, Mervyn.'

'Very funny.'

'That'll put them off.'

'I suggested that it could be tough—'

'OK, OK,' I interrupted, 'we need to keep going. So, Alice, how can we help?'

'I've set up a weekly feedback/wellbeing meeting for them: 2 p.m. on a Tuesday. The more of us that can attend, the better.'

The work Alice did with the trainees was remarkable. By the time it was over, many of them didn't want to leave ICU. We got better trainee feedback during Covid than we had received for years. I think the crucial decision we made was to lead from the front. It is always tempting to stand back, stay strategic and offer advice, while letting the trainees get on with the hands-on medicine. In normal life this is often appropriate, but for Covid we decided that we should be in the bays with the trainees getting our hands dirty, day and night. If we were asking them to risk their own health, then we needed to do the same. This was not a disease we could manage on the telephone from a restaurant or the golf course (not that either were open any more), and having eight consultants resident with the trainees and nurses every night seemed to do wonders for staff morale. We really were all in it together, even if some of what I said towards the end of a thirteen-hour night shift made little sense.

'Great, and that'll be on Zoom as well?'

'Yup. I'm told that Covid won't affect their training, but . . . we'll see.'

'OK, so any other . . . quick business?'

'Oh, sorry, yes.' It was Alice again, apologizing as ever for being conscientious, 'Quick thing. You might have noticed that there are a lot of people in the coffee room at the beginning of each shift.'

If our office was overcrowded, the coffee room at the ICU morning team brief (when the night team give a summary handover to the day staff) was becoming impossible. Everyone working in both the main ICU and the Pods was arriving in that one space each day at 8.00 a.m. Whilst the world outside was staying at home, we were in danger of creating our own crammed commuter tube carriage right in the middle of a Covid ICU.

'It's a nightmare for Elaine. Half of the nurses aren't scheduled to come to ICU, they are just sent down on the day from other wards that are quiet, and hardly any are ICU trained so . . .'

'Shouldn't we scrap the brief?'

'She has changed it,' Alice continued. 'Split it into smaller ones with social distancing, so please bear with them, be welcoming, and from tomorrow the Pods team brief will be across the bridge.'

'Great. Thanks, Alice.' I was over time. 'That's it. Thanks, everyone, same time—'

'I need to do a three wise people discussion about the man in bed 13 of the Pods, if anyone can stay?' Rik asked.

'I can,' I offered.

'Me too,' added Mervyn.

18.03 hours (not bad), and people were shuffling from the room, some clutching a bottle of beer. The pub has always played a vital role in medical staff wellbeing, but the pubs were closed by now, so we'd opened one. 'The Covid Arms' was a pop-up, social-distanced bar that shifted location between the anaesthetic department coffee room and the ICU consultants' office. It served Corona beer and occasionally dodgy white wine (to people not on clinical duties) and was draining our consultant fund, but a drink after these consultant meetings (or sometimes during them) seemed to make the world a more tolerable place.

'So,' Rik began, 'I want to talk about Haydar, who's just moved into recovery, do you both know him?'

'Give us a quick recap.'

'One of our first admissions, sixty-eight-year-old man, background of diabetes, hypertension, but living independently, day twenty-six of symptoms, admitted to us nineteen days ago. Two days of CPAP but struggled, so intubated seventeen days ago. Was proned for a week, very hypoxic but easy to ventilate, and had a nasty pressure area on his face from his endotracheal tube holder. For a while he seemed to improve, but when we started to lighten him up and get him breathing, he deteriorated dramatically. He is now up to 90 per cent inspired oxygen, and his lungs have become very stiff. We've started antibiotics for a possible secondary infection, he's needing high dose noradrenaline and steroids for shock and he's gone back into kidney failure. The questions for today are: should we continue? If so, should we support his kidneys again with the filter? Should we set other ceilings? CPR? And should I get the family in?'

The prognosis for ICU patients depends on their diagnosis, their baseline health (a combination of chronic illnesses, functional capacity, frailty and age) and the number of organs that are failing. Haydar was not old but not young; he had some chronic health issues but was living an independent life and was nearly three weeks into his ICU stay. He was in established severe three-organ failure – four if you included the fact that his guts had stopped absorbing the food he was receiving via a tube, and he was getting worse. It didn't look good. Should we go on putting him through this? He was sedated at the moment, but at best he'd need months recuperating, retraining his respiratory muscles, sleepless nights, delirium, pain, paranoia – torture. For what? What were the chances of him recovering at all, let alone to a meaningful quality of life? Slim, we all thought, but we didn't know. Our opinions were all based on previous experience with other pathogens. We'd never seen this situation caused by this virus.

From another perspective, was he a good use of resource? Not just equipment but people – nurses, physiotherapists and pharmacists. Would they be better deployed looking after a younger, less sick patient with a better chance of survival? We were not rationing officially, of course. We could accommodate more patients, we had space, but every time our numbers expanded the care was thinned, the staffing ratios stretched. So the risk of harm increased, for everyone.

'What do his bloods show?' Mervyn asked.

There was some evidence emerging that certain blood parameters were markers of poor outcome. Persistently low lymphocytes (the white blood cells that fight viruses and produce antibodies) and a high C Reactive Protein (a blood marker of inflammation) seemed to be associated with a bad outlook, but it wasn't binary. It was just another piece of the jigsaw. Haydar's blood markers were not too bad. Not great, but far from the worst we'd seen.

'God, I hate this disease.'

Rik was speaking for all of us, the whole country probably.

'OK, so let's try to be logical.'

I was aware that our mood might affect our judgement. Compassion fatigue is a condition characterized by emotional and physical exhaustion leading to a diminished ability to empathize with or feel compassion for others. Symptoms include lowered concentration, numbness or feelings of helplessness, irritability, lack of self-satisfaction, withdrawal, aches and pains. I haven't had all these symptoms, but at some point or another I have had most of them. Patients who remain critically ill for a prolonged period, despite our best efforts, can leave us feeling helpless, frustrated and irritable. If we are not careful that can soon progress to feeling despondent and hopeless.

The opposite is also a risk. We can become too involved emotionally and be unwilling to let go. We get to know patients, or more commonly their families, intimately over the weeks and months. We become invested in their stories and can lose objectivity. Like them, we start to cling to any glimmer of hope.

The aspiration is to carry on caring without losing objectivity. We shouldn't switch off, be cold and despondent, but neither should we put people through invasive, painful and prolonged treatments that are ultimately futile.

'He's in multiple organ failure,' Rik summarized, 'he's not twenty, he's been here for nearly three weeks and he's getting worse not better. Do you think he's going to get out of here? Home I mean.'

'No.' Mervyn and I replied in unison.

'But,' I added, 'I wouldn't stop.'

'Me neither,' Mervyn agreed.

'He lives independently,' I continued, 'he's not that old, his bloods are OK, he has had a fluctuant course and has a potentially reversible disease. Again, the truth is that we just don't know.'

'OK, yup, fair enough.' Rik was typing a précis of the discussion on to the electronic record. We'd need to review all these decisions in the future.

'And restart the filter?'

The decision was not just 'continue or stop' – often we

draw lines in the sand. A patient might be suitable for a trial of CPAP, but not intubation and ventilation. Each treatment carries a different burden, and the fact that another level of organ support is required may act as a marker that the outlook is now hopeless. Years of experience and data have helped us make these judgements, but it is never 100 per cent. People still surprise us.

'I would,' I said, 'unless the family are saying he wouldn't want this.'

The family's opinion, or more precisely the family's opinion of the patient's opinion, can be key. Most commonly people have not expressed a view. Most of us don't really want to contemplate being on ICU, but increasingly people have made their wishes known. There are problems. Knowledge of our future selves is not always reliable, because, to use an extreme example, the quality of life acceptable to a twenty-year-old has usually changed by the time they are seventy, but if people have made their wishes clear, or even better signed an advanced directive, our decisions can be much easier. However, barring a legal document, these decisions remain ultimately ours. Families can challenge our position, legally if required, but we must weigh up all the information and do what we think is in the patient's best interests.

'I've asked. His family think he would want this. They want us to try everything.'

'I would too, if he was my . . .' he was too young to be my dad, but too old, in my head, for a brother, 'relative.'

It has become my benchmark, my sense check. What would I do if it was my brother, sister, mother, father, wife or child? It doesn't always help. Sometimes I still don't know and I just end up feeling more depressed, but it feels like a good test of the decision's rigour. I don't know if it means I make better decisions. I am anxious and unsure by nature, a worrier, and maybe this just makes me more likely to put off making difficult decisions. 'Carrying on' is often the path of least resistance, but that doesn't mean it's the right one. Perhaps it drives my colleagues mad, when they take over from me and are left to pick up the cans I've kicked down the road, but I don't deliberately shirk difficult decisions and I'm not going to change. At least this way I can justify the decisions to myself, even if to no one else.

'CPR?' Rik asked.

Mervyn and I both shrugged. It was a question that had to be asked, but also in many ways was academic.

'If it's something quickly reversible, yes. If it's the end point of a gradual decline, no.'

'Great, thanks, guys.'

'We should review it, though, regularly,' I said, spotting a flicker of doubt on Rik's face, 'If things change.'

'Or don't.' Mervyn added, gloomily.

As I left the changing room that evening I bumped into Jamie coming in for a night shift.

'Hey, how's it going?'

'Night shift.'

'Ah, sorry. How have the nights been, for the emergency "family"?'

'Mixed.'

'Do you get some sleep?'

'On a trolley in the toilet.'

'What?'

'We're sleeping in the toilet, on the second floor.'

'Why?'

'Because that's where they've put us.'

'Who's they?'

'The people who hate us.'

'*In* a toilet?'

'Not in . . . it's a changing room, with a toilet in it. People come in though, in the night, to use the toilet.'

'Nice.'

'Not to . . .'

'I've got to go, Jamie. I want to catch the kids. Sleep well.'

A few days later we admitted Jonathan, a slim, thoughtful forty-year-old. He had been diagnosed with leukaemia in December 2018 and initially treated with chemotherapy, but the leukaemia had relapsed, so on 20 March 2020 he'd undergone a bone marrow transplant to knock out the cancer once and for all. His new bone marrow (donated by a sibling) had engrafted successfully and begun to produce cells, but Jonathan had suffered a series of complications and was still in a weakened state when in the second week of April he caught Covid. Soon after that he came down to ICU for CPAP. He responded well to the positive pressure, his oxygen levels improved, and his breathing settled, but from the start I was preoccupied by what we should do if he progressed and required ventilation. The outlook for leukaemia patients who require intubation and ventilation on ICU is poor compared to other groups, and Covid could only worsen those statistics, but on the other hand Jonathan was officially cured of his leukaemia. He might be weak and still dealing with the complications of his transplant but he was also forty, with a wife, Megan, and young children.

Although I am suspicious when people talk about 'fighting' diseases, I have to admit that from the outset Jonathan looked like a man in the heat of battle. He sat upright in his bed, often gripping the sides, and was fully focused on the task at hand. He knew that if he ended up on a ventilator his outlook was bleak so he was doing everything humanly possible to avoid it. He had a family to get home to and half his life to live.

I spoke to Jonathan's haematologist to confirm that the bone marrow transplant had indeed been successful, but I didn't need to have a three wise people discussion. If he progressed to the point of requiring sedation and ventilation, that's what we would do. Like Jonathan, I was just hoping desperately that it wouldn't come to that.

5. Public Response

6 April 2020

'Tom! Are you coming to watch this?'

'In a minute.'

'OK, well, it might be over in a minute.'

'Just gonna finish this game.'

Tish, Edie and I all stared at the TV. Tom was lying on his back halfway up the stairs, headphones on, legs plastered up the wall and fully immersed in a game of Fortnite on his Switch.

'Good evening,' Huw Edwards began as the music faded. 'The prime minister, Boris Johnson has been moved to the Intensive Care Unit of St Thomas' Hospital for closer observation . . .'

'When are you on?' Edie asked, her attention already sliding back to a YouTube video on her phone.

'I don't know. Next? He *is* the prime minister.'

'Can I have something to eat?'

'What would you like?' Tish asked.

'Toast?'

'Just wait till Dad's bit, and then I'll get you something.'

A picture of St Thomas' Hospital flashed up on the screen.

'Thank God they took him there,' I mumbled.

'Can I have a snack, just while . . . is that your hospital, Dad?'

'No. Grab yourself a biscuit and get me one.'

Edie leaped to her feet and scuttled out of the room.

'The move is said to be a precaution,' a reporter told us from outside the hospital. 'The prime minister is described as being in good spirits, but . . .'

'Blimey, do you think he's going to die?' Tish pushed herself to her feet and set off towards the door.

'Where are you going?'

'Loo.'

I looked around the deserted room as Huw moved on to the next item.

'Now, tonight Fergus Walsh, our medical correspondent, sends us an exclusive report from inside one of London's busiest intensive care units.'

'I'm on!' I called.

'Coming,'

'Can you pause it?'

'No.'

'Do you want a tea?'

'NO! Just come and share in my discomfort.'

Tom ambled into the room.

'Dad, can I get a computer? Not just for gaming, but I've seen one . . . Oh is that you?'

I'd been on TV twice previously, to my knowledge. In 2003, during a brief stint as medical advisor to *Holby City*, I was asked to play a non-speaking anaesthetist opposite a glamorous and very much speaking surgeon. Unable to respond verbally due to a lack of Equity membership and talent, my replies to her questions consisted of gurns and frowns. To say they were unconvincing is to be generous, and almost all were cut from the final edit. My right shoulder, however, was superb in the back of one shot, and the day was not completely wasted, as I did eventually pluck up the courage to speak to the surgeon (using actual words) off camera. I was not brave enough to invite her on a 'date' (she was off the telly for goodness sake) but I had a plan. I was working at GOSH at the time, and they regularly had celebrity visitors to cheer up the children, so I invited her there.

It turns out that children don't really watch *Holby City*, but one or two parents vaguely recognized her (with prompting) and smiled politely. She gave out some signed scrubs for an hour or so, and then we beat a hasty retreat to Ciao Bella across the road. Three hours later we were the last to leave the restaurant (even the piano player had packed up and gone), and three years later we were married.

A few months before our wedding, I was on call when Alexander Litvinenko died in UCH ICU. I'd only been a consultant for a year and the whole experience was unsettling and stressful, not least when I was asked to give a statement to the press. I'd already spoken to his wife and son, so at about 10.30 p.m. I set off downstairs to deliver some pre-written words to a group of journalists in the central reservation of the Euston Road. The police had redacted several sections of the statement, meaning that the remaining words jumped across the page unevenly, and that, combined with some last-minute advice to 'take no questions under any circumstances', did little to settle my nerves.

I stumbled through the piece, doing a good impersonation of a reluctant six-year-old in the school nativity, but eventually made it to the end and was about to leave when one of the journalists, who was all of two feet in front of me, said, 'Sorry mate, I couldn't hear a word of that, could you just . . .'

'No questions,' I barked, already on my way back to the hospital. This hospital spokesperson (as I was later labelled on *Sky News*) was not falling for any of their journalistic trickery. Fortunately, the timing meant that few people saw this performance, but Tish not only watched it, she also offered some constructive criticism.

'The thing to do,' she suggested when I got home, 'is to read through the statement before you say it out loud. That way you can convey the sense of it.'

'Thanks, darling.'

This time it was going to be different. I was older and wiser, and there was an important message to get across. The curve had to be flattened, we needed people to follow the lockdown and stay at home.

Fergus and his cameraman, Adam Walker, visited us on Friday, 3 April. It was a tough day, particularly for Elaine, because it was the day we admitted our first nursing colleague to ICU. Tricia was a youthful sixty-year-old with short blonde hair and a refreshing no-nonsense attitude. She'd decided to become a paediatric nurse after doing a bank shift at GOSH during her training and after forty years spent working largely at that one institution (her home from home) she'd risen to the position of head of nursing for Haematology and Oncology. Usually she commuted to work from the family home in Broadstairs, but for the previous two weeks she'd been working especially long hours and staying in a hotel in London. She was a key part of the effort to clear beds at GOSH in order to make room for children from other hospitals which in turn needed all their beds for Covid. In the last few days of March she'd started to feel unwell and on 30 March tested positive for Covid. By 2 April she was breathless and came into UCH. Hours after that, she was moved up to ICU for CPAP. She was stoical from the outset and responded well to the CPAP. It was time to watch and wait.

The BBC planned to speak to our clinical director, David, matron Elaine and, because I was on for the Pods, me. David would speak about operational issues, Elaine about the staff and patients, and I would talk about some clinical aspects.

We began in the seminar room, where I showed Fergus our wall map of ICU and explained the process for labelling and managing beds. I began to relax. I seemed to be able to get a sentence out at least, and Fergus was nodding encouragingly.

The response at home was less respectful.

'Thanks for teaching us our colours, Dad,' Edie offered sarcastically as she munched through a third digestive.

'Purple for Covid,' Tom was now doing an impression of a nursery school teacher, 'blue for . . . ?'

'Non-Covid,' Edie offered.

'Very good, Edie. Have another biscuit.'

'Hilarious,' I muttered.

With the first set of interviews completed, we set off to don our PPE and enter the clinical area. The donning station of the Pods, where we deposited valuables including phones and put on our PPE, was at the entrance to the theatre complex, but the patients were a further 20 metres down a corridor in the recovery areas. Sorting out the camera equipment was taking time, and I was getting twitchy about doing a ward round on camera, so I decided to go ahead and recap on the state of the patients before Fergus, Adam, Elaine and David joined me.

The Pods had been open less than two weeks, and it wasn't just the anaesthetists who were struggling to work in them, it was everyone. Apart from the fact that it was hot, crowded, windowless, isolated and full of critically sick patients, it was also nobody's 'home'. The anaesthetists and theatre nurses were used to the physical space, but it had been transformed beyond recognition. A lot of the equipment was new, and much of the old had been repurposed. They'd used the anaesthetic machine ventilators for years, but not on sick ICU patients for days on end. It turned out that our particular machines needed to be recalibrated every twenty-four hours or they'd revert to the most basic form of ventilation, which was wholly inadequate for Covid patients. Someone had to hover, poised by the bedside at the dreaded moment each day to switch them back on to a decent mode. No one had seen that coming. And the anaesthetists and theatre staff didn't know the cadence and rhythms of the ICU day. That was the remit of the ICU nurses, but they were out of their usual environment using machines they'd never seen before.

Added to that, the two groups did not know each other. They didn't know each other's seniority, skill sets, strengths and weaknesses or personalities. They had all been thrown into this melting pot of Covid ICU without a clear idea of how it would work. Was that a consultant or a brand-new SHO? Or a nurse or a physio? Should the ICU nurses do what the anaesthetists said or should they question them? Where did the responsibility lie?

The buck stopped with us, the ICU consultants, but some of us were not anaesthetists and so were equally unfamiliar with the environment. And some of us turned up for a ward round at 9.00 a.m. sharp, while others were off at meetings until halfway through the morning. It was impossible for the teams to plan, because every day it all changed. The anaesthetists felt frustrated, the nurses voiceless, and the atmosphere was in danger of becoming toxic.

Having listened to both groups, the solution seemed to be for the ICU consultants to sort themselves out and for Elaine to decamp to the Pods, so I tried to bring a level of consistency to the way our group worked, and Elaine donned PPE. For ten days she immersed herself in the Pods. She fetched and carried, drew up drugs, made suggestions to the anaesthetists, answered questions, spotted problems, supported staff who were struggling and brought in assistance, and gradually the teams came together. It didn't solve everything – we still had a growing number of very sick patients, different kit every day and a disease we didn't understand – but it re-empowered her nurses and averted what could have become a major crisis.

At first it was strange to have the microphone and camera darting around the bed spaces on the ward round, and we felt exposed and self-conscious, but very soon we forgot they were there and were barking information and instructions at each other through our PPE as normal. There are no quiet asides when you are in a mask, hat and visor.

One solitary patient was awake. Taken off the ventilator the previous day, she was a slight, late-middle-aged woman who was still very weak and welded to a CPAP mask. Most of the day she kept her eyes closed, but I don't think she was sleeping. She was just shutting out the horror of her environment and situation. Each time I approached her bedside I felt guilty. I didn't want to disturb her and force her to engage, especially with a large man dressed in a space suit. I thought her decision to withdraw was very reasonable, but I had to check she was OK, so I took her hand gently in my double gloves. She didn't respond. I needed to introduce myself, but speaking was useless, she'd never hear me, so I shouted.

'Hello, Geraldine.' I shook her arm slightly. 'Geraldine, I'm Jim, one of the doctors.'

She opened her eyes, nodded and closed them again. She was not up for a chat, but she was OK. Her breathing pattern was good, her other systems were working independently and each day she was able to do a little more with the nurses and physio-therapists. I talked through her parameters with the team; blood results, nutrition, bowels, kidney function, confirmed the plan for the next twelve hours and then leaned forward to offer her some encouragement. Again it felt uncomfortable to shout at such a small, vulnerable woman, but I tried to be as gentle as I could.

'You are doing well,' I said, 'going in the right direction.'

She nodded slightly, but she didn't open her eyes.

'We're pleased.' I let go of her hand. Normally I'd ask if there was anything she'd like to ask us, but she was giving no indica-tion that there was, and she'd struggle to let us know through the CPAP mask, so I turned to her nurse. 'Anything else?'

'No, I don't think so, thank you.'

'Family up to speed?'

'Yup.'

Apart from an hour for lunch and a couple of quick coffee breaks, ICU nurses spend the whole twelve-and-a-half-hour shift with their patients. In normal times it means that one nurse spends all day with their one patient, so the relationship is intimate and intense. Often they return to the same bed shift after shift. If the patient is unconscious, then part of that relationship is transferred to the partner or other family members, who can be almost living at the bedside. When a patient starts to wake up and is delirious and disorientated, the nurse at their bedside is their lifeline. They are completely vulnerable, reliant on this one person's skill and compassion. The best nurses know everything about their patients, medical and non-medical. Often they write a list of the patient's likes and dislikes on the wall:

LIKES	DISLIKES
Arsenal	Orange (flavour and colour)
David Bowie (pre 1985)	Being referred to as 'Geoff'
Pointless	The One Show
The Today Programme	Gardener's Question Time
Monty Python	Spurs
Raspberry yoghurt	Jazz

They might also write up a daily regime, something to give the longer-term patients structure and purpose as they increase their strength over the days and weeks. They work out what makes that particular patient tick; a new grandchild, or the dream of a long-planned holiday, whatever it is that makes the struggle worthwhile. And they are skilled clinicians. They spot deviations: subtle changes in the physiology, a rash on the back since starting the latest antibiotics, a change to the sleep pattern or the ECG or the patient's affect. This was truer than ever in the Pods.

So for the doctors to come on the ward round and make plans without consulting the bedside nurse is unforgivable. Having said that, I have done it, more times than I care to admit. It is so easy to get tunnel vision and ignore other people's perspectives, particularly when you are under pressure or unsure. It is a strange paradox that often the more we need to consult, the less inclined we are to do so. Asking for help and opinions when you are the boss is not always easy, but it is vital. There are many facets to each patient, and a single clinician is bound to miss things. Checking with the nurses, physios, patients and relatives reassures me that I've done my best to cover everything. In a strange way it is also a barometer of how well I am doing the job: the more I am listening, rather than speaking, the better. I am relieved to say there is no official tally of my performance, but the occasions when I've got it badly wrong stick painfully in the mind. I remember as a registrar perching on the bed of a patient who'd just undergone major surgery.

'What I'd do,' I began confidently, 'If I were you is—'

'What I'd do,' he interrupted, 'if I were you, is not sit on a patient's bed without asking them. It hurts.'

I can still remember the shame as I slunk off the side of his bed, desperately avoiding eye contact with his wife. How many other patients have wanted to say the same, but been too anxious or polite or felt too vulnerable and reliant on my help to do so?

When we finished the ward round, Fergus kept the camera rolling and took Elaine and me aside to ask us a couple of follow-up questions. For a second I worried that inadvertently he'd reveal a gaping hole in my medical knowledge which would be spotted on TV by, amongst others, an eagle-eyed member of the GMC, who'd feel obliged to bring my career to a rapid and public conclusion in a desperate attempt to restore public confidence in the NHS at such a crucial time, but I needn't have. Fergus, as always, was courteous and patient, and I was on safe ground: it was Covid, no one knew the right answers. I was just starting to relax again, when I overheard Elaine thanking her husband for his support. The pandemic was not easy for the families of frontline workers, and mine were (deep down) incredibly supportive, so I thought it would be nice to thank them too, publicly. I was completely unprepared for what happened next. As I talked about Tish and the kids my face started to feel hot, but it wasn't the PPE. And then my voice cracked, and my eyes filled with tears.

'Oh Christ!' I thought, 'keep going, keep going, faster, get through it, maybe no one will notice,' but by the time I finished with 'and I am just incredibly grateful to them' I was barely getting the words out.

'Are you crying?' Tom asked, incredulous.

'No.'

'You are, you're blubbing,' Edie confirmed.

'It was . . . a long day. I think I'm a bit allergic to the masks.'

'Yeah, right!' Tom giggled.

'Daaaaad!' Edie was now squirming off the sofa with embarrassment.

'What? I was, you know . . .'

'You only had us so you could look good on TV.'

By now Tish was laughing too, but she gave my hand a squeeze and said, 'Ahh, sweet.'

I was genuinely surprised to become so emotional talking about my family on camera. Like many key workers, I'd wrestled with where to live through the pandemic. Should I be going home every night, potentially taking the virus with me? Tish, Tom and Edie were low-risk, as far as we knew, but what did that mean? It didn't mean no risk, and I'd seen young, fit people become extremely sick and die. I am not a brave person, but I wasn't going to stop working. I am not old, I can still run round the Heath, and we had good PPE, so there was no excuse for me to avoid the hospital, but I didn't have to expose my family.

With lockdown looming, they could have relocated to Tish's parents' farm in Kent, like evacuees in the war. I had visions of an idyllic isolation spent collecting eggs, baking cakes and running through the fields with dogs, but I would have missed them all terribly and am very grateful they stayed. We did talk through the options, but we couldn't even work out how they could isolate from me long enough to avoid posing a risk to Tish's vulnerable parents. Then lockdown arrived, and it all seemed a bit late. Briefly, we discussed me staying in a hotel, but again we had no idea how long it was going to go on. I might be there for months and turn into Alan Partridge. I asked a few colleagues what they were doing, and they all shrugged:

'Just sort of carrying on.'

'I'm not allowed into the house without a shower.'

'I feel a bit guilty about my mother-in-law. She doesn't come out of the basement so much any more.'

To treat myself more than anything, I set up a regime. I kept my phone, keys and wallet in a plastic bag at work and wiped them down at the end of the day. I showered after each shift, even washed my hair, and usually wiped down my bag, but not always. I gelled my hands incessantly, sometimes wiped surfaces before putting down my computer and tried to turn down offers of crisps from other people's packets.

Tish was supremely relaxed. She accepts and deals with risk in a way that I can only dream of and was more than happy for me to come home each night, as long as I contributed to home schooling. And we were lucky. We still had an income, we have outdoor space, friendly neighbours and a Heath within five minutes upon which to exercise the dog, me and the children. Like the rest of the country I missed my extended family, my parents and siblings particularly, but I saw them most weeks on Zoom.

The reaction of the public was extraordinary and confusing.

I missed the first three weeks of clapping because I was working, but for the fourth I was at home. I emerged tentatively on to the front doorstep, unsure as to whether I should clap or accept the applause from other people, but of course they weren't applauding me. They were clapping for all the key workers, and not just the key workers, for all of us, for sticking to the rules and flattening the curve. I am not an epidemiologist, but the effect of the lockdown seemed obvious in the hospital. I am convinced that the willingness of the public to follow these measures saved thousands and thousands of lives and prevented the hospitals from being overwhelmed. The emergence of the public on to their doorsteps every Thursday evening to wave, smile and clap our general determination seemed a lovely thing. I felt part of a community, surrounded by kind, generous people who were looking out for each other. Many of my neighbours are no longer spring chickens and have been shielding. They must have felt frightened and isolated at times, but every Thursday without fail they appeared in their front gardens with pans, lids and spoons to bash together.

Inevitably the children took a different view. One week of clapping was just about fair enough, but every week? By the time I got to join them for this heart-warming event they'd moved on – to sarcastic clapping.

'Time for your clapping, Dad,' they shouted up the stairs, before shuffling out through the front door to slouch against a tree. Each individual clap they managed, seemingly a huge effort, was followed by a sigh or yawn and a long look at the time. After a minute or so they were asking if 'they could go now' and soon after that they were flat on their backs, barely stirring.

At the time I pretended to complain about their lack of gratitude, but the truth was I enjoyed their irreverence. They understood how serious the virus was, they got the sacrifices that people were making and they missed their grandparents desperately, but they were not going to let their Dad get away with thinking he was some sort of hero who deserved weekly clapping.

Tish's reservations were more political.

'This is not a substitute for ten years of underfunding. The nurses need paying properly, not clapping,' she hissed, clapping heartily and then whooping at the horns of passing cars.

On 23 March I received a message from a paediatrician friend.

'Mad celebrity mates Damian and Helen want to organize pizza delivery to ICU – is this helpful?'

'Yes it is!!' I replied immediately, adding 'the Lewis-McCrorys?'

'Yes. Pizza should be coming your way.'

I knew that Damian Lewis and Helen McCrory lived in North London and for some reason I assumed that they were going to arrive on our unit in person, perhaps in motorbike leathers with a huge box of pizzas; it was a strange time, and nothing surprised me any more. I even prepared my best *Homeland*, *Band of Brothers* and *Peaky Blinders* chat (one of which I've actually seen), but of course they didn't come. They did send pizzas, though, which were delicious, and then with Matt Lucas went on to set up 'Feed NHS'. Then more pizzas arrived – and curries, and fresh bread and sushi, and salads and mini burgers, and teriyaki – every day from large chains, smart hotels and local restaurants – mountains of it. Some of it was donated for free, some paid for out of funds raised by the general public for NHS staff.

When I qualified as a doctor people told me that I would be so flat out and caught up in the work that I wouldn't even think about food. Many newly qualified doctors, they assured me, missed two, sometimes three meals in a row when they were on call before they even noticed. This worried me, because I am not good without food, but it needn't have. In the twenty-six years between then and Covid I have never forgotten about a meal and I have never missed one. There is always time to eat.

So thank you to all those who donated food (and money for food) during the pandemic. This doctor for one was extremely grateful and did his absolute best to eat it all.

Having said that, I did catch myself, a few weeks in, leafing through the pile of meals in the staff room, grumbling,

'Urghh, is there nothing apart from pizza and curry?'

'There's sushi,' someone offered.

'Try the risotto, it's great.'

'Nah, I really fancy Chinese.'

I hadn't bought myself lunch for over a month and I was on the verge of becoming a spoiled brat.

It wasn't just food that people sent in. The desire to donate was insatiable. Companies sent boxes and boxes of clothes (mainly underwear and pyjamas), toiletries, fold-up beds, wine, cash, hampers, gift vouchers and fobs for exclusive underground car parks. Every day was like Christmas in Matron's office. The generosity was touching, but also at times troubling. All these donations came from shops that were shut, restaurants, cafés and hotels that couldn't trade and in the case of my car-parking space, a film production company that was paralysed. We, in the NHS, had jobs. We were going to work, receiving pay packets and were secure in our professional futures. It wasn't fun, but our lives were continuing to a certain extent as normal. It occurred to me, as I walked down a deserted Tottenham Court Road to work one day, that we were the only place still functioning. Everything else was closed. Quickly typed notes filled the windows of every shop and café.

'Closed for the foreseeable future. Hope to see you soon. Keep safe.'

Rows and rows of them were all a variation on the same theme. I was pleased that London was so empty. In my mind's eye I could see the virus searching the deserted city for its next victim and being thwarted, but it was eerie. On some days it seemed that only empty buses roamed the streets with a lonely, masked driver at the wheel. How many of these businesses would ever reopen?

When the bombs went off in London in 2005, some friends of mine from the West Country cancelled a trip to the city. It wasn't worth the risk, they said, too dangerous. I was shocked. The bombs were horrifying, but I live in London and I didn't feel scared. Perhaps I did for a day or two, but after that we all just carried on and went about our business. The next bomb could be anywhere in the country, in the world. After 9/11, however, I did cancel a trip to the States. I knew that it was illogical, but something made me fearful about flying to America. I think things seem more frightening sometimes if you are outside them, and the further away you are, the scarier they become.

I was stressed and I was fearful. I am not claiming that Covid didn't frighten me. Like almost everyone I was waiting to get it, expecting at any moment to develop a fever and a cough and take to my bed, so I used three mantras to try to rationalize it:

Statistically, when/if I catch Covid I should be OK.

I could be hit by a bus tomorrow.

None of us is getting out of here alive.

But I wasn't really falling for any of them. At times through the peak I was relaxed and fatalistic, but at other moments I was tense and tetchy, particularly at home around the family. I snapped at Tish and the children about social distancing and following the rules, when I'd no reason to suspect they weren't, and I justified my behaviour by reminding myself that I'd been working hard at the coalface, seeing the worst Covid could do, things that they couldn't possibly understand. More likely, I was just tired, anxious and a bit scared.

★

At 9.00 p.m. that night, 6 April, I sat down in my study for a Zoom meeting with the 'cons rota admin' WhatsApp group. Alice had put the group together three weeks previously to do just that, consultant rota administration, and at the time I'd groaned at the prospect of yet another festival of Whatsapp tedium, but it turned out to be just the opposite. The group consisted of Rik, Alice, Steve and me. We had some Zoom meetings, worked out the rota and then had a few more to check that it was working and to deal with sickness and teething problems. It became clear that we worked well together, and it felt as if four was a good number for Zoom meetings, so soon we were organizing meetings whenever one of us was grappling with a problem and wanted some fresh ideas.

Rik was the engine. He knew everything that was going on, went to all the high-level official meetings and acted as our fount of all knowledge and information. Alice was the conscience, always thinking about how any ideas we had might impact other groups: the nurses, trainees and colleagues; Steve was the innovator, approaching each problem from a slightly unexpected angle and often unearthing simple elegant solutions; and I was the experience. Every time they came up with an idea I sense-checked it against the previous fifteen years on ICU.

We didn't make decisions. David was the boss, and the consultant meeting was our decision-making forum, but we did come up with a few ideas and proposals. And then over the weeks the group gradually morphed into something else as well.

'Hey, Jim.' Rik was first on the call. As ever, he was sitting in front of a clothes horse of drying pants. Often he had his five-month-old baby on his lap, but tonight he appeared to be Zooming solo.

'Hi, Rik, all right? Hi, Steve.'

Steve always Zoomed in from his loft conversion and seemed

to have at least three screens open at all times, judging by the way his eyes flitted around the camera.

'Hi, guys.'

'Is Alice – oh, hi, Alice.'

'Evening, everyone. Sorry, just saying goodnight to the girls.' Alice had decided in mid March to send her two older children to stay with their cousins on the Isle of Skye for the pandemic, leaving herself and her husband (a consultant anaesthetist at the Royal London Hospital) with only their thirteen-month-old baby. Initially the girls had been delighted, but two and a half weeks in they were missing Mum and Dad and starting to get a bit cross and very homesick.

'All OK?

'Yeah, yeah, just guilt, you know, the usual.'

'It's an adventure,' I suggested, but as I said it, I realized it was exactly what I'd come up with the last time she was having a wobble.

'That's what I . . . anyway. So?'

'It was your idea to Zoom, wasn't it, Alice?'

'Sorry, Rik, yes. Sorry, right.' Alice cleared her throat, 'Couple of things. Some good news first. There are five consultant intensivists from GOSH who want to come and help us.'

'Help us?' Steve queried.

'Work with us, do shifts. They're twiddling their thumbs and want to get stuck in.'

'That's amazing.' I had not been expecting this. 'I mean fantastic, not surprising . . . anyway . . . great.'

'So the question is, what do we want them to do?'

'My night shift on Wednesday?'

'How much adult ICU have they done?' Steve asked. 'Just because I'd be fairly useless on a paediatric ICU.'

'It's easier going from children to adults than vice versa,' I asserted confidently, based purely on my own personal abject fear of looking after small children.

'Do they want to join our rota?' Rik asked, before pressing mute, picking up a small child from between his feet, taking her out of the room and rejoining us.

'I think they'd have to be extra, but . . .'

'We can't expand our rota,' Alice interrupted.

'Day shifts, on the main unit?'

'I guess, to begin with.'

'They've offered to do nights.'

'DAD! CAN YOU BRING UP MY BOOK AND A WARM MILK AND BISCUIT?'

'I'm on a call . . . haven't you brushed your teeth?'

'I'M HUNGRY.'

I pressed mute.

'Have an apple.'

'THEY TASTE HORRIBLE AFTER YOU'VE BRUSHED YOUR TEETH.'

'So you have brushed . . . can you ask Mum?'

'MUM!'

'Sorry, guys,'

'You're on mute, Jim.' I pressed unmute.

'Sorry, sorry. The children have completely stopped going to bed.'

'So we've got a proposal for the GOSH consultants. I think they will end up doing nights as well.'

'Amazing!'

'DAD, WHERE'S MUM?'

'She's gone for a walk.' I pressed mute again. 'You're supposed to be asleep. OK, have whatever you want.'

I unmuted.

'When will they start, Ali?' Rik asked

'Couple of days.'

'Great.' I paused, but no one spoke, so I grabbed my opportunity. 'Are any of you guys taking Vitamin D?' I'd meant to get a straw poll of consultants earlier in the day.

'No.'

'Why do you ask? Do we look deficient?'

'Mervyn's convinced that Vitamin D deficiency is a risk factor, he's measuring all the patients' levels on the unit.'

'You still taking hydroxychloroquine, Jim?' A smile crept across Steve's face.

'I never actually took it.'

'I think you're confusing him with Donald Trump.'

I felt my face redden. Back in March I'd come shamefully close to starting myself on prophylactic hydroxychloroquine. At the time it had been presented as a cheap, well-established drug that had theoretical anti-viral properties and might either treat or prevent Covid. Like Donald Trump, I'd fallen for it. A trial in healthcare workers was being proposed, but I'd thought, sod that, if it might help, why not just take it? Fortunately, Dave Brealey publicly pointed out that I was being an 'idiot', because there was no evidence for the drug (except that it had side effects) and so I backed off. At the time of writing, hydroxychloroquine has been shown to be of no benefit as a treatment for Covid, and no evidence has emerged of its use as prophylaxis.

'Not my finest hour,' I admitted, 'but I do think Vitamin D is different. It's harmless, and apparently there's some data from somewhere . . .'

'I've heard Mervyn talk about Vitamin D,' Rik agreed, 'but I think he's just on his hobby horse.'

'All right,' it was clear they were going to be no help on the Vitamin D question so I moved on. 'One other thing, are you wearing facemasks? I mean out and about.' We were still months away from any national guidance, and masks were very much the exception around London.

'Not really. Occasionally.' Rik muted and then spoke expressively to someone off screen, shrugged, smiled and returned to the call.

'They don't make any difference, do they?' Steve also seemed uninterested.

'They make people give me dirty looks.' Alice is of Korean heritage and was already sensing hostility in the street even without a mask. With one, she was clearly up to no good.

'The China Virus.'

'Trump!'

'Piss off.'

'Can we talk about the trainees?'

'Sorry, Alice, of course.'

And so the conversation went on. We talked about the trainees and then drifted on to a couple of patients, until at 10.30 Steve yawned, glanced at his watch and made his excuses. Within a couple of minutes we'd all dispersed to apologize to our spouses.

We always met to discuss a particular problem that one of us was facing, but increasingly we used the Zooms to talk about work, life and the pandemic in general, and by the first week of April I realized that Rik, Steve and Alice had become my Covid work family. I don't know their real families well, I've never been to any of their houses and before the pandemic I wasn't particularly closer to them than other colleagues, but through the crisis I began to rely on them more and more. We saw eye to eye, they were always on the end of the phone when I needed them, but most importantly I trusted them.

When something was bothering me, I told them. Whether it was a patient, a government diktat, a clinical strategy, Vitamin D or just a sense of hopelessness about the future. If it was troubling me, I raised it at a 'cons rota admin' Zoom call. The group emerged organically and disintegrated again as the crisis ebbed.

It wasn't formal, it was just four people throwing around ideas and listening to each other's Covid anxieties and, of course, marvelling at Rik's collection of pants.

On Easter Sunday morning Tish and I decided to cycle with the kids to the centre of town. We are not a great cycling family. Tom particularly tends to wobble precariously and should ideally not be too close to traffic or water when on a bike, but this weekend we decided to go for it. It was another beautiful day, so we set the alarm for 6.30 and, after some minor grumbling, biked down through Kentish Town, Chalk Farm, Primrose Hill, Regents Park, Regent Street, Haymarket and Trafalgar Square. We turned right through Admiralty Arch into the Mall and continued up to Buckingham Palace. The whole way we hardly passed a motorized vehicle. Bicyclists were spread across the Mall (not just Tom) as if the city was closed to cars. We chatted to other families, ate a sandwich and then turned left down Birdcage Walk, through Parliament Square and up to Downing Street. Still the streets were deserted, and we paused outside the famous gates. I thought we could use the opportunity to discuss the politics of the day, perhaps the timing of lockdown and whether there was any chance left of avoiding a hard Brexit, but the conversation turned out to be more practical.

'Can we go home now?' was the only question Edie wanted answering. So we did.

It was on days like these that Tish and I wondered if something good might come out of all of this. There were no planes in the sky, no cars on the road, the air was clean, birds were singing, even the bees seemed to have a fighting chance – perhaps we could return to a better normal.

6. Peak

9 April 2020

One advantage of getting older is that I find it easy to nod off in the afternoon. Before a night shift this is a useful skill. I'd gone to bed at four and set the alarm for just before six so that I could dial in to the evening SitRep meeting and get an idea of what was going on. My shift started at eight.

The ICU was full (thirty-five beds), the Pods had a further twenty-one ventilated patients, and up on the CPAP unit there were another eighteen. The patients were getting sicker. Only two had recovered and been discharged to the ward since my last day shift two days previously, and three had died. We'd taken three in from other hospitals that day, we were taking roughly five per shift from the Emergency Department, and the last non-Covid patient had been moved out.

'OK, thanks everyone, that's it for today.'

I pushed myself out of bed and threw on a T-shirt and a pair of jeans. I barely bothered getting dressed for work these days, it was straight into scrubs when I got there.

Downstairs Tish was making food, while the children sat listlessly at the kitchen table. They were not feeling well. It was the Easter holidays, three days until Easter itself, but none of us had really noticed.

'Pasta with salmon?' Tish asked.

'Have you checked their temperatures?'

'Yes. Normal both of them.'

'You're not coughing are you, guys?'

'Edie's got a migraine, and Tom's got a tummy ache. Does that sound like Covid to you?'

'No, no. Pasta with salmon sounds lovely.'

'I'm going to bed,' Edie stated.

'Dad, we're not coughing.' Tom's head flopped on to the table with weariness.

'I thought you said kids don't get Covid?' Tish handed me a bowl filled with steaming hot, creamy salmon pasta. She looked tired and worried.

'No, you're right. I don't think they do really. Thanks.'

There wasn't the slightest indication that either child had Covid, but at the time any hint of illness in the family set off a series of alarms in my head. It must have been exhausting for Tish and the kids.

'Sorry,' I added.

'Don't worry, it's nice that you care. Well, nice-ish.'

My new year's resolution had been to bicycle to work more often, but at the start of the pandemic that plan had gone out of the window. The exclusive underground parking space I'd been offered off Charlotte Street was too good to pass up. As I wound my way around the car park's tight turns, I started to plan my night. I'd get a handover from the day duty consultant and then quickly check in with the different areas to work out the hot spots – I stopped.

There was a car in my designated space. I say mine. Obviously it wasn't mine, it belonged to the friend of one of my colleagues, but nonetheless I felt affronted. There was one other spot free, but it meant some tricky tight reversing, and as I turned sharply to squeeze into it I heard the miserable scraping of metal on metal. What possible purpose could a red metal post be serving there? I took a deep breath, pulled forward, realigned and slipped back into the space.

It was another beautiful spring evening; Tottenham Court

Road was deserted, and for a moment I felt calm, ready to take on the night. Then I remembered the car. I hadn't inspected the damage, maybe it wasn't as bad as I'd thought.

As I walked into the hospital, I passed Jamie going the other way.

'How was the day?' I asked.

'The day was OK.'

'But?'

'No, it was fine. I went out with the transfer team to the North Middlesex. Blimey, if you think we've got it bad.'

'What do you mean?'

'Half their staff are off sick and there are patients everywhere.'

'You brought someone back?'

'They clapped us out the door.'

'I bet you loved that.'

'No . . . well, a bit maybe.'

'How's Vuppe?'

'Nightmare!'

'Burned her paws on the underfloor heating again?'

'She's been to the vet four times in the last three weeks.'

'Why?'

'The first time she just sort of faded.'

'Faded?'

'She had a chicken leg, we think, or some drugs possibly from Camden and then she just . . . *faded*. I was up all night sitting with her, and she went floppy and kept closing her eyes.'

'In the middle of the night?'

'So Sammy took her in first thing the next day.'

'What did they think? Chicken leg or drugs?'

'The vet looked in her mouth and stuff and seemed to think she was OK.'

'Sleeping at night is OK, then?'

'But then on the way home, she started chewing weirdly.'

I was biting my cheek now.

'Chewing what?

'Something she'd picked up, so Sammy took her back.'

'Oh my God! And . . . ?'

'They were very nice about it.'

'Promise me you two will never have children.'

'And then we started worrying about the fifteen pugs next door so we had her spayed.'

'I think Sammy needs to get off furlough as quick as possible.'

'Oh God, and before that she jumped in the river and started vomiting so we . . .'

'She's a dog, Jamie.'

The difficulty with taking handover as the night consultant was that five different areas were all handing over in different places at once. The Pods, the two different halves of the original ICU, the CPAP ward and 'the rest of the hospital' were all huddled in different rooms, passing on the details about their patients. During the day there'd been four different consultant intensivists covering these five different areas, but at night there was just one. There were lots of other doctors around, highly skilled ones, a respiratory consultant and several consultant anaesthetists for a start, but there was only one consultant intensivist. I was the only person in the hospital who in normal times ran an ICU so at handover I really needed to be in all five places at once.

Prior to Covid my last night shift was in January 2005, at the Royal London Hospital. I'd waved goodbye to them forever I thought, without a single ounce of regret. I found nights draining, stressful, lonely, and invariably I slept badly in the daytime. My lowest point came on Christmas morning 2002, when I was halfway through a gruelling run of seven night shifts and found myself sitting on the sticky floor of the ICU coffee room eating my Christmas 'treat' of watery scrambled eggs out of a plastic kidney dish designed for urine collection. I might be back doing night shifts at nearly fifty years old, but at least the catering had improved.

'Hi,' I said, pouring myself a coffee as Steve wandered into the office.

'Where are the hot spots?'

'Hmm,' he replied. 'It's all fairly hot, I'm afraid.' Steve was the daytime duty consultant, meaning that he'd been holding the duty phone, managing referrals and helping out wherever needed. He'd been busy.

'OK.' I was determined to stay upbeat. 'Should I get handover from you or . . .'

'The other guys are coming, except Rashan, who's handing over the Pods in the anaesthetic coffee room.'

'OK.'

'Out and about, there's two you need to see straight off on HDRU. Ronan just called. They're both three days into CPAP and not thriving. Oxygen's up to 90 per cent. Sorry, I'd have gone up, but I've been donned in the Pods helping with a ventilation issue.'

'No problem.'

'They're making beds for those two. The question is whether you tube them upstairs or bring them down then intubate them.'

'Gotcha.'

'Oh, and one of them's a healthcare assistant.'

We both paused and looked at each other.

'Not from here?'

'No.'

A few minutes later, the two consultants from the main unit joined us and began to brief me on all the areas of most concern. It was impossible to get a detailed handover of everyone, but they tried to prioritize the problems while I scribbled everything down on my piece of paper, circling the issues I needed to deal with first. I couldn't get to the theatres handover as well, so I decided to let that go. I'd start my night ward round there, once I'd been up to the HDRU to see the two on CPAP and then regroup and work out where to go next. The anaesthetic consultant joining me on the main ICU that night was Pete. He is not an intensivist, but he should be. I spent a year when he was a registrar trying to persuade him to do ICU, but he was having none of it. Too sensible, perhaps, but he was doing it now, and he'd definitely cope until I could get there.

'Call if anything doesn't make sense,' Steve shouted over his shoulder as the door slammed behind him. None of it made sense.

I popped my head into the anaesthetic department coffee room to reassure them I'd be round the Pods as soon as possible and then set off up to the HDRU. It was the first time I'd seen it transformed and filled with CPAP patients, and it was impressive. The lights were low, and there was a sense of quiet calm and competence, but the first patient I saw worried me. She was a large woman in her late fifties, with a receding jaw. The CPAP mask was strapped tight to her head, but air leaked out constantly. She was sitting up with her head thrown back and her eyes closed. Her breaths were steady, but she looked exhausted and as advertised she was on 90 per cent oxygen and barely maintaining her oxygen sats. She needed a ventilator, but her size and receding jaw suggested it might not be an easy intubation. To anaesthetize and intubate her on the ward, with limited equipment and expertise, would be risky. On the other hand, the transfer down in the lift without a tube in her precarious condition was far from risk free. If she decompensated en route, it would be a nightmare.

'If you could get her things together, we'll take her down and tube her on the unit.' I confirmed to the nurse at her bed space,

'There's another one, a healthcare assistant, sorry I've forgotten his name, also on 90 per cent oxygen.'

'Yes, Ray, bed 18.'

I made my way down the hushed corridor to bed 18. Ray was younger, late forties and awake.

'Hello,' I said. 'My name's Jim, I'm from ICU. How are you getting on?'

'OK,' he replied, but he needed another two breaths before adding 'tired'.

I glanced over at his CPAP machine. He was also on 90 per cent oxygen and breathing thirty-five times a minute – too fast. He needed a ventilator, too, but perhaps not quite as urgently.

'OK, Ray, we'll take you down to the ICU very soon. Just bear with us.'

Ray nodded.

'I think we may well need to pop you off to sleep and take over your breathing for a while, but we'll get you downstairs first, is that OK?'

'Sure.' Ray closed his eyes.

I never know what language to use with patients who are fellow health-care workers, or any patients for that matter. Does the word 'pop' make it all sound less terrifying and more run of the mill, or is it just patronizing and irritating?

I remember as a medical student listening to my GP trainer request that a patient pop up on to the couch, pop his pants down and pop over on to his side so that she could pop a finger into his back passage. I couldn't tell if it was reassuring or a bit sinister. Sometimes I think I should be professional, respectful and slightly distant, but my natural disposition is to be a bit chummy, and so usually I revert to that. I hope that it dissipates some of the tension, particularly in an anaesthetic room before an operation, but I'm sure that sometimes it just adds to the anxiety. People don't always want their doctor to be their best mate.

The time I definitely get it wrong, though, is when I let my irritation show. About six years ago I arrived to see Clare, a patient of roughly my age about to have an operation for breast cancer. She was due to be first on the list and so, having gone through my usual set of questions and explained our plan, I added, almost as an afterthought, 'And you've not eaten or drunk this morning?'

'Oh, yes, I had breakfast at five thirty, as per my letter.'

She smiled, but, rather than smile back and reassure her, I clenched my teeth and frowned. The day was now a shambles. Patients should be six hours without food before an anaesthetic to allow the stomach to empty. Once anaesthetized, with the protective reflexes obtunded, food in the stomach can reflux up the oesophagus and down into the lungs, causing pneumonia. None of the other patients could go first for various reasons and now, because she'd had breakfast, neither could Clare. We'd be sitting twiddling our thumbs for the first three hours of the day and then run over beyond our 7 p.m. scheduled finish, and I'd miss the kids.

'Sorry,' she added.

'No, no. Not your fault,' I managed, but I wasn't convincing. I am terrible at keeping my emotions off my face. Did she not know that you shouldn't eat before an operation?

It turned out that she'd been perfectly entitled to have breakfast because originally she'd been booked into theatre for the afternoon. It also turned out that she was a film producer, who blogged through her illness; the blogs were then continued by her brother when she got too sick to write and eventually, after she died, turned into a brilliant, funny and heartbreaking book called *Not That Kind of Love*. She wrote about the day of her operation: 'I felt like I was back at school and the teacher had given me that "I am so disappointed in you look" when your homework came back covered in red marks.'

I felt awful when I read it, but I learned a lesson. It is so easy to ignore a power imbalance when you are the person with the power. Autonomy is often inadvertently removed from patients, particularly when they are vulnerable, lying on their back on a trolley, waiting for an operation. As health-care workers we should do everything we can to be mindful of that.

On my way out of the CPAP unit I called the ICU registrar, Ato. Ato is unfussy, a man of few words (around me), but what he does say is invariably worth listening to.

'There are two up on T7 that need to come in. Can you let the nurse in charge know? They're both CPAP, confirmed Covid, but sick – on 90 per cent. And can you call the intubation team? Are you happy to do the transfers?'

'Sure.'

'Thanks Ato, bring them on CPAP, usual Covid transfer precautions, I need to go round the Pods, but call if you're not happy.'

'Will do.'

As I wiped down and put away my phone I felt guilty. Perhaps I should bring them down myself. Having made the decision to transfer them unintubated, was it fair to ask someone else to do it? Ato would be just as safe as me, he's extremely capable, but was he really happy? I was his boss – not just a boss, his personal educational supervisor. I would be writing his assessment at the end of the placement. It would be a big call for him to question my decision. I glanced at my watch, it was ten o'clock already. I needed to get round the Pods and then the main ICU. I'd made my decision: he was competent to do the job, and I couldn't be everywhere at once.

As I made my way down to the Pods, I checked my phone.

No missed calls, thank goodness, and just one text message from Edie.

'Dad I have just woken up and can't sleep again. Tom is sleeping in your bed mum has been AMAZING. I love you x.'

'Love you too x,' I replied.

One of the biggest changes to ICU practice during Covid was the inability to 'nip' in to a patient to have a quick look, pass on some information or ask a simple question. Intensive care patients change all the time. Although we set plans twice a day, between times things happen: blood results come back, specialists visit, and patients 'go off'. When this happens, we nip in, reassess, chat to the nurse at the bedside and alter the plan. In Covid each 'nip in' meant a whole fresh set of PPE and five to ten minutes of donning and doffing. The result was that visits to the bedside were far fewer, and while each one missed had only a minor impact, the cumulative effect was significant. When we did put on the PPE it was important to get as much done in that single visit to the bedside as possible, so we'd collect up tasks like a shopping list before entering the Covid zone. You were either in getting clinical work done and cut off from the outside world, or out catching up with admin and having a break.

Nowhere was this more the case than in the Pods. The geography meant that, having donned, we walked 20 metres down a theatre corridor to the patients, accompanied only by the noise of our own breathing within the mask and visor. It was a few moments alone to reflect. That night I remember being struck by how much this simple corridor, like the world, had changed. Once a bustling theatre thoroughfare, it was now just a dimly lit, deserted conduit to our new makeshift ICU. No one had operated in any of these twelve theatres for nearly three weeks and wouldn't again for who knew how long.

The Pods had expanded since I'd last been here: new patients, new and unfamiliar equipment, new staff and they'd spilled over into the paediatric recovery and a pre-operative waiting area. There were twenty-one patients in total, all Covid, all sedated and ventilated, six turned on to their fronts and five on filters. This isolated, claustrophobic, temporary unit alone was now far busier than the majority of ICUs in normal times.

I pushed open the double doors and was relieved to spot Kirstie, one of the anaesthetic consultants, on the other side. Kirstie is a head and neck anaesthetist, so used to managing sick patients with difficult airways for complex twelve-hour tumour surgery. She is not an intensivist, but she had volunteered to become one for Covid, and as well as being supremely competent, she is a mate – this ward round was going to be OK. As we went from bed to bed, most of my job was to listen and agree. She and her colleagues had seen all the patients, plans were in place, and the nurses were comfortable with what they were aiming to achieve. Two patients had been moved over from the main ICU earlier in the day, but they were already settled, and Haydar was back on the filter but otherwise stable. There was the odd ventilator to adjust, fluid balance to review and drug regime to tweak, but generally things were under control.

By 12.30 we'd seen everyone in the Pods, and my visor was giving me a headache, so I thanked Kirstie and the team, who were going off for a well-earned break, peeled off my PPE and picked up my valuables. I'd missed a couple of calls from Pete, whom I'd abandoned on the main ICU four hours earlier, and one from Ato.

'Please, not the transfers,' I muttered to myself as I hurried back across the link bridge to the main unit.

Ato was waiting for me when I arrived back at ICU reception. He looked calm, but then he always looks calm.

'All OK?' I asked innocently. 'Sorry, I've been in the Pods.'

'Yeah, A couple of things . . .'

'Transfers?'

'Fine, both down. Trudy is tubed in bay 1 and Ray is in bay 4 still on CPAP.'

'Great, brilliant, thanks. You're a star.'

He looked at me quizzically.

'No problem. Are you OK?'

'Yeah, yeah fine, thanks for bringing them down.'

'There is one in ED I need to talk to you about, though.'

'Sure, just let me catch up with Pete and I'm all yours.'

I slumped into a chair behind the main reception desk. This 12 foot by 12 foot alcove was right at the heart of the ICU and the centre of everything. Three SHOs sat at computers along the back wall, typing up notes, while Pete finished a conversation with one staff nurse and two others packaged specimens to be sent off down the chute to the lab. A month later we'd limit the number of people allowed in this cramped space, but for now it was bustling with people and activity.

'Pete, sorry, I abandoned you, how's it going?'

'OK-ish.'

He sounded far from convinced.

'Go on.'

'No, we're all right, there's a few we need to go through. Bay 4 is a bit of a nightmare, but we're getting there.'

'Can I hear from Ato and then . . . ?'

'Yup, absolutely. Give me a shout when you're done.'

I was torn. Pete was not happy, but he is a consultant, so I turned back to Ato.

'We brought one up from ED about an hour ago. Fifty-nine years old, duck. He's in bed 5 on CPAP. They're just putting the lines in, but he's settled for now on 55 per cent oxygen.'

'OK. Is that our last side room?'

'No, one more, and one who could go round to the Pods, so we're OK – for now.'

'Great.'

'But I've just been called about a woman in ED with acute kidney injury.'

'Right.'

'Not Covid, but she is a bit complicated. Nineteen years old, history of inflammatory bowel disease, had a liver transplant and a colectomy last year. Fever, high stoma outputs, and her potassium's 8.'

My heart sank.

'Syrie Constable?'

'Do you know her?'

I'd not met her, but I knew her history, and I knew her father. He is the brother of a friend of mine from medical school, and we'd had several conversations over the previous week.

Since the age of twelve Syrie had suffered with auto-immune hepatitis, a disease in which the body's own immune system attacks the liver. She'd been treated with various immune suppressants, but progress had been slow, and just when the liver eventually did start to improve in 2016, she developed inflammatory bowel disease (another auto-immune disease causing severe bowel inflammation). The combination proved extremely difficult to treat. By late 2018 she had to stop attending school and through 2019 spent 260 days in hospital. The only option left was liver transplantation, and in November 2019 Syrie received a new liver. At the same operation the surgeons removed part of her spleen and some inflamed bowel and brought the end of the remaining bowel out through the wall of her abdomen to form a stoma. Her recovery was slow because she'd been so weakened over the previous year, but she made it home for Christmas. The surgery was a success, and at last she could look forward to a brighter future, although, like all transplant patients, she would require lifelong immunosuppression to stop her body rejecting the organ.

In March 2020, however, she developed fevers and high fluid outputs from her stoma. Her team thought that a reactivated virus in her bowel, able to proliferate due to the immunosuppression, was the most likely culprit, but investigations were ongoing, and in the meantime she was in and out of UCH with fevers and dehydration.

On 3 April her father phoned me. He was terrified. She'd been in again for a few days, dehydrated with a sky-high temperature and barely functioning kidneys, but it wasn't her illness that worried him, it was Covid. If she caught Covid, there was a high chance she'd die.

Initially they'd put her in a side room on a Covid-free ward. The staff were dealing only with non-Covid patients, and it felt relatively safe. Her parents' visiting was limited, but they were getting in to see her enough, and the plan seemed cogent. The number of Covid cases, however, was rising quickly, and soon the ward Syrie was on was having to take them, so they moved her to a different section; a new side room in a Covid-free area. On 3 April, however, the bed managers had no choice but to put a man with suspected Covid into a bed less than 15 feet from Syrie.

There was still a closed door between Syrie and the man, but the nurses were going in and out. They could easily pick it up from him and take it in to her. What should her father do? Kick up a fuss? Call the chief executive? Call the press? He was grateful for the care and didn't want to get any staff into trouble, but this was his daughter. He felt surrounded, trapped. She wasn't well enough to go home, but equally not safe in the hospital. Syrie had been through so much over the last six years, but finally she'd had the prospect of getting her life back, taking her A levels and going on to university, and now this.

I remember sitting on the stairs at home with my head in my hands. What could I say? I'd have felt the same way. They deserved to be kept safe and looked after in a Covid-free space, but there wasn't one. Even if the other patient didn't have it, who was to say that the staff weren't carriers. None of us was being tested.

On balance I felt that Syrie was in the safest place possible. Each time anyone entered or exited her room they'd wash their hands, change gloves and put on a mask and apron. It is second nature for health-care workers and none of the other patients would come close enough to be a threat. There weren't any better, more secluded side rooms available, so her father and I agreed that she should be vigilant about infection control and move only if and when a safer bed became available. The next day she was moved back to a Covid-free ward and a few days after that she went home. She'd got through a nine-day stay in our Covid-filled hospital without catching it, but now two days later she was back, with a potassium of 8.

A normal potassium level in the blood is between 3.5 and 5.5 mmol/L. Above 6.5 it can cause potentially lethal heart arrhythmias, so a level of 8 needs urgent intervention. In normal times, once they'd given emergency measures in ED, I'd have brought Syrie straight to ICU for ongoing treatment and monitoring. Her potassium level was life-threatening, but for Syrie so was Covid, and our ICU was full of it.

'They don't want to send her here, necessarily,' Ato continued. 'They just wanted to check you're happy with their plan.'

'She's had dextrose and insulin and calcium?'

'Yeah, yeah.'

Insulin drives the potassium into the cells and calcium stabilizes the heart. They would control things in the short term.

'OK.'

'They've got a room. Isolated. They can put her on a monitor, put an arterial line in and keep an eye.'

'Potassium of 8, though. It's very high.'

Ato looked thoughtful.

'ECG's normal, and she's very dry. They're pouring in fluids, it should all settle . . .' he tailed off.

'OK, yeah.' I looked up at Ato. 'Well, better than bringing her here, I guess.'

By now I really was guessing. It was another Covid compromise, except that Syrie didn't even have Covid.

'I'll pop down, just to check she's OK.' I added.

'Don't go too near.'

I spent the next twenty minutes running through some issues with Pete and then I set off for the Emergency Department.

It was deserted. I entered through the 'Majors', section where rows of cubicles, usually occupied noisily at this time of night by the party-goers of Soho and Camden, were empty. The lights were low, and small huddles of doctors and nurses tapped quietly on computers, as if trying not to disturb each other. The party-goers were at home, presumably watching telly, but where were the heart attacks and the strokes? I walked on past 'Resus', behind the waiting room and through into the urgent treatment centre. I'd never seen the department like this. Rows of seats were unoccupied, punctuated by one lone drunk, snoring peacefully. Staff hovered restlessly at the nurses' station. The contrast with upstairs could not have been greater. I knew people were trying to avoid hospitals, but I hadn't expected this. It was unnerving. Were people so scared of catching Covid in hospital that, however ill they felt, they'd rather take their chances at home?

Finally, I arrived in the Emergency Assessment Unit (EAU). Designed as an overnight facility for patients who may or may not need admission, the EAU is a busy, acute unit usually brimming with patients. That night I could see two.

'Hi,' I said, catching a staff nurse's eye. 'Sorry to bother you, I'm from ICU. Have you got Syrie Constable down here?'

'Over there.'

She pointed to a bed space on the other side of the unit with the curtains three-quarters drawn. Through the gap I could see a tall, young woman with long, dark hair sitting up in her bed. I made to wave and then stopped myself. I wanted to go over to talk to her, but I knew I couldn't.

'How's she doing?'

'Better. She's passing urine, and the potassium's down to 6.5.'

'Great.'

'We've got a side room for her, with a monitor. Do you want to see her?'

'No. No, it's fine, thank you. I don't want to . . . lots of Covid upstairs.'

'OK.'

'Is her dad still here?'

'Went home about half an hour ago.'

'OK. Well, look, call us if you need anything.'

'Sure.'

I looked across at Syrie again. She was lying back now, straightening out her sheets and chatting to her nurse.

'You OK?'

'Yeah, fine. Thanks. Better get back.'

Syrie was discharged home from EAU two days later. She never needed to venture deeper into the hospital and yet again she avoided Covid. The EAU team made a brave decision and did a fantastic job.

When I arrived back on the main ICU, I was directed straight to bay 2. Julie, the nurse in charge of that area, needed help. Out of her five patients, three were acutely unstable.

The lights were low in the bay, and through my visor everything looked fuzzy and indistinct. It was stifling, and the air felt heavy. I don't know why, perhaps I was just exhausted, but each breath felt like an effort, sucking the mask into my lips and then blowing it away again.

Julie was with Ravi, a man in his fifties who'd been with us for five days. He'd come in breathless and been put quickly on to a ventilator, but over the last twenty-four hours he had started to develop multiple organ failure. His temperature and heart rate were up, his blood pressure was down, and his kidneys were starting to fail. He'd had an echocardiogram (a scan of his heart) during the day shift, which had confirmed that it was starting to fail, particularly the right side, which pumps blood to the lungs. Visions of Adam went through my mind. We needed to get on top of this quickly, but it wasn't straightforward.

'Hi,' I said, glancing up at Julie as I felt Ravi's feet. Even through two sets of gloves they were icy cold.

Julie was attaching a syringe to the bottom of eight infusion pumps at the back of the bed space.

'Jimbo. We need a plan. The BP keeps crashing. I've given 500 mls of fluid, but he's stopped responding.'

I like Julie. She's sharp, Scottish and irreverent and she lives life to the full. She's always just been somewhere or is planning something that sounds both exciting and exhausting. Tonight she looked harassed.

'OK,' I began, 'Norad's on?'

'15 mls of double strength.'

Noradrenaline or 'Norad' is a drug that constricts the blood vessels. When people have sepsis (or severe inflammation), the blood vessels dilate and become leaky, causing the blood pressure to drop. The mainstays of treatment are fluids and noradrenaline, but neither help a heart that is failing.

'The Doppler shows . . . ?'

'Stroke volume's rubbish.'

The Doppler is an ultrasound probe which sits in the gullet and measures the size of every heartbeat, the stroke volume. If it is too low, the two options are to give more fluid to fill the heart more or give drugs to make it pump harder.

I fiddled with the Doppler probe that was sticking out of Ravi's mouth and looked at the screen. Julie was right: the stroke volume was best described as rubbish.

'Enoximone's on?'

'Four, but when I go up, the pressure drops.'

This made perfect sense. In addition to the noradrenaline, Ravi was on enoximone to make the heart pump harder, but unfortunately it also dilates the blood vessels so can drop the blood pressure.

'OK, blood gas?'

'On the computer.'

I picked the small piece of paper off the computer keyboard and ran through the numbers. The blood was acidic, and the potassium up to 6.9.

'And the temps still up?'

'38.3.'

'Right,' I took a deep breath, 'I think we need the filter and GIK. Titrate the Norad to a pressure of 60 and the GIK to a cardiac index of 2.5. Give some calcium to get him on to the filter. Let's start some bicarb as well and get cultures. Oh, and watch that temperature. I presume he's already on antibiotics?'

I looked up. Julie had stopped what she was doing and was glaring at me.

'What?' I asked, taken aback.

She spread her hands, looked around the bay and shrugged. I followed her eyeline. A few small PPE-clad figures shuffled around the bed spaces.

'You're bloody joking, Jim!'

'Sorry, I . . .'

'It's just me. You know that, right?'

I looked again at the other staff. I didn't recognize any of them. These were not ICU nurses, they were ward nurses, helpers and medical students. They couldn't set up the filter or draw up complex, powerful infusions, or interpret the cardiac output monitor. GIK is made up of three different infusions: glucose, insulin and potassium. It is novel and clever but also labour-intensive and hazardous. Get it wrong, and you might cause the potassium to go life-threateningly high or the glucose brain-damagingly low.

'That guy needs a filter too, by the way.' Julie pointed at the patient behind me. 'He's acidotic, and his potassium's climbing, but I've only got one, and, like I said, there's only me. Unless you're going to set this filter up and manage the five patients while I go hunt for another one.'

'OK,' I mumbled. I hadn't got the first idea how to set up a filter.

As I tried to come up with a more realistic plan, one of the ward nurses slipped a piece of paper with another blood gas result into my hand. I glanced down at it.

'Oh my God, whose is this?'

She pointed to a man lying on his front on the other side of the bay.

'OK.' I looked again at the small piece of paper in my hand. 'All right.'

Julie folded her arms and waited.

'Sorry,' I said, forcing myself to look her in the eye.

I'd got this badly wrong. I wasn't helping, I was just adding to her problems. Normally there'd be four or five trained ICU nurses in this bay by now and two or three doctors. With three acutely unstable patients, this would be the focus of the unit. All spare staff would be here, drawing up drugs, running through lines, setting up filters, taking samples and collecting equipment. We would sort out all the problems at once, in parallel, but not tonight.

ICU is by its nature unpredictable, so we are used to busy nights. It is not uncommon for me to come in at three o'clock in the morning to deal with an emergency, and 'firefighting' shifts are a regular occurrence, but this was different. We didn't just have a handful of critically sick patients, we had sixty of them, and we'd run out of nurses and equipment. I needed to rethink my whole approach. I'd messed up and in the process upset one of our best nurses. We could no longer work in parallel. I needed to prioritize the problems, simplify and set up a workable plan.

'Right,' I said, trying to think logically, but my mind was still racing. 'OK, so forget all that. Let's start on adrenaline.'

'Great.' Julie had re-engaged. 'Rose, can you get me one of the pre-filled adrenaline syringes? Eight milligrams in 50 mls.'

Adrenaline is the second-hand Land Rover of heart stimulants. It's old-fashioned, dirty and rough around the edges, but also powerful, reliable and it does everything. It stimulates the heart and tightens the blood vessels and so increases both blood flow and blood pressure. This was what Ravi needed right now. It can also cause unstable heart rhythms and worsen the blood acid levels, but those were risks we'd have to take. Julie had syringes of adrenaline ready to go.

'So who needs the filter first?' I continued.

'Ravi,' Julie replied, already connecting up the adrenaline syringe. 'We've got a bit of time next door, I think. Potassium's only 6.4 and he's not too acidotic yet. Not passing urine, but . . .'

'OK,' I turned to the nurse next to me. 'Rose?'

'Yes.'

'I'm Jim, hi. Sorry you're a . . . ?'

'Staff nurse, from the Emergency Department.'

'Great, thanks, that's great. Could you run through some dextrose and insulin for this chap?' I pointed at the bed behind me. 'And we'll need a 1.26 per cent bicarbonate infusion, 70 mls per hour, as a holding mechanism.'

Rose nodded. These were treatments she understood.

'I'm going to deal with the carbon dioxide in bed 20.'

The piece of paper I'd been handed was the arterial blood gas of the patient opposite Ravi. He was a man in his sixties, whom I'd never met before, but it was a familiar story – diabetic, smoker, high blood pressure, Covid, very bad oxygen levels, blood pressure support, hard to ventilate, kidneys holding on for now.

An arterial blood gas is a bedside test that tells us the oxygen, carbon dioxide, acid, electrolytes and haemoglobin levels in the blood. In the sickest patients we run them every couple of hours, more frequently when we need to, and then adjust our treatments accordingly. The alarming thing about this man's blood gas was his carbon dioxide (CO_2). At 25 KPa it was five times the normal level. The blood carbon dioxide level usually relates directly to ventilation: the more you ventilate the lower it goes. When we have a panic attack and hyperventilate, our carbon dioxide drops, and we feel giddy. By breathing in and out of a paper bag we breathe back in our own carbon dioxide, allowing it to build up in the blood again, and we feel better. He had the opposite problem. We couldn't ventilate him enough to clear his carbon dioxide because his lungs were so stiff.

We allow the carbon dioxide to rise in ICU because we don't like to ventilate the lungs too hard, but as it rises it makes the blood increasingly acidic, and at a certain point this affects the function of the other organs. A carbon dioxide of 25 KPa was too high.

As I tweaked and twiddled with the ventilator opposite, Julie rescued Ravi's blood pressure and then successfully connected him to the filter, and Rose stabilized the third patient. We were almost back running in parallel. I popped back and forth between the bed spaces, checking on progress and offering help and advice, and fifteen minutes later we were joined by an SHO, who re-sited a line, prescribed some medication and fluids and caught up with documentation. We were working as a team again, and gradually things started to improve. Ravi's blood pressure came up, I made some progress with the carbon dioxide, and we sourced a second filter.

An hour and a half later, with a plan in place, Julie was relieved for a break, and the two of us pulled off our PPE and left the bay.

'Sorry again, about that . . .' I mumbled, searching the box for my bag of valuables.

'That's all right.' Julie grinned, 'Idiot.'

Pete was already at the main reception when I arrived. I glanced at my phone. It was 4.30 a.m.

'Sorry, Jim,' he began.

'What? Why?'

'I gather you've been busy in bay 2.'

'Don't be ridiculous, how are 4 and 5?'

This was typical Pete, always playing down what he'd been up to and apologizing for not doing more.

'The nurse in bed 33 needs a tube, I think.'

'Ray?'

'No, he's in 31. We've already intubated him. Tricia.'

'Oh no. OK.'

Having two colleagues on the unit was upsetting and disconcerting for the staff. These were fellow frontline NHS workers, people they might have trained with or worked alongside on a bank shift in another hospital. They were also clinical staff who had become critically sick with Covid. Had they caught it from patients? Had they been exposed to a particularly high dose because of the nature of their work? Had they used the same PPE as us? No one verbalized this, the nurses continued to work as professionally and compassionately as ever, but these questions crossed my mind, so I assume they crossed theirs too.

Tricia, the head of nursing from GOSH, had coped well on

CPAP for four days, but her oxygen requirement was increasing now and she was starting to get tired.

'OK, let's call the intubation team, and I'll join them. Have you spoken to her family?'

'Not overnight.'

'Do you mind giving them a call?'

Tricia was still calm and focused but she was exhausted, and there was no more she could do. It was time for us to take over, and she knew it. As the intubation team assembled their equipment and carried out the checklist, I knelt by her bed, took Tricia's hand and ran through the plan. She gripped my palm and nodded as I tried to reassure her, her eyes trained on the ceiling above her head. I explained that we'd spoken to her family and would do so again once she was asleep and safely on to the ventilator. I promised we'd look after her and then stepped back to let the intubation team do their thing.

Dan and Max were ice-cool. They'd performed a lot of Covid intubations by this time (this was their third of the night) and had developed a slick and almost silent routine. Dan delivered the drugs, while Max gave oxygen and calmed the patient. When Tricia was asleep, Dan began the timer, and Max gently ventilated the lungs with a bag and mask. Sixty seconds later Max slipped his video laryngoscope into the mouth, and manoeuvred it until a view of the vocal cords came up on the screen. There were secretions at the back of Tricia's mouth, so Max picked up the suction catheter, inserted it alongside his laryngoscope and cleared them to improve his view. The note of the oxygen saturation bleep started to fall, but Max seemed oblivious. Calmly he picked up his endo-tracheal tube, deftly moulded it and slipped it into the mouth. The back of Tricia's mouth was crowded and fitting the tube past the laryngoscope was awkward, but after a couple of attempts its tip appeared on the screen. Max advanced it towards the larynx, but it butted against the front of the vocal cords and would not advance. I felt my fingers twitch and glanced up at the monitor. The oxygen sats were now 80 per cent. Max, seemingly moving more slowly the more pressure he was under, pulled back his tube and advanced it at a different angle. Again it got caught, so he withdrew and twisted it. The oxygen sats were now 72 per cent, and with every bone in my body I wanted to shout: 'GET ON WITH IT!'

But I forced myself to keep quiet. Shouting at him was unlikely to help.

This time the tube slipped through the cords.

'Stylet out please,' he requested quietly, but he needn't have. Dan was already leaning forward to withdraw the metal stylet from within the tube so that Max could push the tube itself down into the trachea.

The oxygen saturations were 50 per cent, but the tube was in, and within a couple seconds Max was ventilating the lungs. Soon the oxygen levels had begun their slow, painful ascent.

'Great, well done, thanks guys,' I said as if I'd never been worried. 'I'll set up the vent.'

'No worries. Any more intubations?' Dan asked.

'Hope not.'

Finally, I made it back to the consultant's office at 6.45 in the morning. It was a bright, sunny day outside, and light streamed in through the gaps between the blinds. I looked at the folded camp bed and the limp pile of pale blue NHS blankets. I wondered if it was even worth setting it up as I picked a fresh packet of digestives from the box. I was starving. I never miss meals, but I'd eaten nothing all night.

I pulled open the bed, poured myself a glass of milk, took three digestives from the packet and lay down, but I didn't sleep. I lay staring at the ceiling with the night's patients whirring through my head. How long was this going to go on? How much worse would it get?

At 7.10 the door opened, and my colleague Rashan's head appeared.

'Oh no, sorry, Jim, sorry to disturb you.'

'No, no. Don't worry, I'm not sleeping. Come in.' I beckoned.

'I brought you a tea.'

'Thank you.'

'How was the night?'

'Umm, well . . . you know.'

'Good news. You remember Fadi, the young guy with the café, who we sent to Queen Square?'

'Yeah.'

'Doing great, wide awake, off the ventilator.'

'No way! That's amazing, Rashan.' I could have hugged him. 'Will you put something round the group, to let everyone know?'

'Of course.'

It wasn't until three days later that I noticed the large, dented, red streak down the passenger side of the car. The decorative stripe of chrome was buckled and came off in my hand.

'What kind of person would do this and not even leave a note?' I grumbled to Tish. And then I remembered.

7. Low Point

Late April 2020

'Hi, hun.'

'Hi, lovely, how are you doing?'

Jonathan took two deep breaths and repositioned himself in his bed.

'They're going to take over.'

'OK.' His wife, Megan was completely calm.

'Put me on to the ventilator.'

'OK. OK.'

Jonathan looked up at me and tilted the iPad in my direction. I leaned forward into the frame to see Megan sitting at her kitchen table.

'Hello, hi . . . It's Jim, one of the ICU doctors. We spoke on the phone, yesterday.'

'Yes, hello.'

'I think we should take over Jonathan's breathing. He's fought very hard, but he's exhausted and . . . I think it's time.'

'OK.'

I tilted the iPad back towards her husband.

'I love you.'

Jonathan pulled the mask slightly off his face so that he could speak more clearly.

'I love you too. And the kids. Give them a big hug.'

'I will. Big hugs, lovely.'

There was a pause, and again Jonathan glanced in my

direction. Each breath was an effort for him now. I swallowed hard and stepped forward.

'So we'll gently pop Jonathan off to sleep and take over his breathing. The team is outside getting things ready now. I'll give you a call afterwards. Is that OK?'

'OK.'

I looked back at Jonathan. He nodded and closed his eyes.

'All right, lovely. I love you,' she continued. 'I'll speak to you soon.'

Jonathan nodded again and passed the iPad back to his bedside nurse.

The intubation team was waiting for me outside the room, donned and ready to go. I pulled off my mask, nodded to them and headed for the sink to wash my hands. I knew that if I spoke, I'd cry. As I scrubbed between my fingers the emotions settled, and, without looking up, I thanked them.

'No problem,' they replied, pushing open the door to Jonathan's room.

I don't know why some patients make such an emotional impact. Perhaps the question I should be asking myself is why I'm not struggling to control my emotions all the time. Why is it that I can do an ICU ward round, talk to two or three families about how bleak the outlook is for their loved ones and within ten minutes be having a laugh in the coffee room about the Christmas party? Why is it that I can anaesthetize a list of cancer patients with complete composure, only to cry my eyes out that same evening over a film about a fictional person dying of cancer. It bothers me. Sometimes I think that I should be more demonstrably in touch with my emotions when it comes to the real patients, caring more deeply. Can I really deliver the best care if part of my brain is worrying about the SHO on nights who's gone off sick?

There is no doubt that good communication is vitally important in medicine. One of the medical defence organizations demonstrated that with a three-day communications course they could reduce the rate of formal complaints against doctors by 50 per cent. Patients really mind how they are told things, but the difficulty is different people want to be communicated with in different ways. Some want professional detachment and clarity and an honest opinion, however hard it is to hear; others, empathy and to be offered any tiny glimmer of hope. Some want to know every detail and option, others just want to be told the best course of action. Perhaps carefully judging that is more important than 'feeling' the patients' pain.

Being distracted by a staffing crisis is clearly not ideal, but it is reality. Everyone has distractions. This is our job, we do it every day, it's messy, and life goes on around it, but I think patients always know whether they have had our full attention. They deserve it, and our time, and we should do everything we can to give them both.

I am aware that we all have good days and bad days, both technically and emotionally, but in darker moments I do wonder how nice I have actually been to patients and families during my career. I am not rude, but I am probably kinder to some than others. I certainly get on with some better than others. I try to make myself imagine that I am in the patient's shoes. What would make this experience less frightening? But I probably do that less often than I should. It's draining. Twenty per cent of ICU patients die, I work in a specialist cancer hospital, and my regular anaesthetic list is for breast cancer. I know that I can't care deeply and personally about every patient. A level of detachment is necessary to survive – without it I would have burned out long ago. I try to judge my conversations and interactions as carefully as I can, but in the end I have to rely on the belief that I am a decent human being, so naturally treat people well in their time of need. I hope that on the whole I do, but I'm haunted by the times I've got it wrong and try hard not to repeat them.

It is odd to admit, however, that I can go through a whole day relatively unperturbed by sick and terrified ICU patients, only to come home and have a meltdown about my son playing computer games when he should be doing his homework.

Then there are people like Jonathan and his wife Megan, who knock me sideways.

Jonathan (the forty-year-old admitted with Covid following his bone marrow transplant) had battled on with CPAP for nearly a week but eventually he became exhausted, and both he and I agreed that enough was enough.

By now we were starting to get some data, and the headline was that nearly half of ventilated Covid patients did not survive. These statistics made every Covid intubation a poignant and sobering moment. We ventilate people every day in ICU, but the sheer volume of Covid patients, combined with the stark statistics and the ban on family visiting, made for a very different experience. So we decided to allow one relative in to visit their loved one in person before the intubation. This might be the last opportunity they'd have to speak to each other face to face, and we felt that that justified the risk. Unfortunately, Megan has asthma and was shielding at home with her children, so together they'd made the very tough decision for her not to visit, feeling they couldn't put her at any risk.

Jonathan had met Megan when they were both working in the theatre industry, she as an associate set designer and he as a lighting programmer. They'd married, had the children (now six and nine), and she'd continued her work in theatre, while he moved on to light big live music events.

I'd spoken to her on the telephone the day before. When Jonathan spoke to me it was through the CPAP mask (and I was in

PPE), so his voice was muffled, and he was breathless and uncomfortable. It was difficult to get a sense of the man, but talking to his wife in her own home with the sound of the kids in the background gave me an insight into his life. I could imagine organizing play dates with them at the school gates, or sitting in the park drinking coffee as our children played football. I'd tried to be upbeat with Megan, to emphasize how determined Jonathan was, and she'd gone along with it, clinging to positives, but we'd both known he was struggling.

At the beginning of the pandemic communication with relatives was incredibly difficult. Each day, after the ward round we divided up all the patients and then telephoned their families. We tried to do this at a set time each day, between 2 and 3 p.m., but inevitably there were emergencies and admissions, and some of the phone calls got delayed. Sometimes that was just for an hour or two, but occasionally they were handed over to the night team, and once or twice they got forgotten altogether. I can't imagine what it was like for relatives, sitting at home, waiting for the call. Many of them telephoned the ICU reception or the nurse in charge, desperate for information, but they couldn't be put through to the bays because the bedside nurses were in PPE and so couldn't answer the phone. There is often a power imbalance in medicine between carer and cared for, but the strict limitation on visiting added an uncomfortable dimension. The last time these people had seen their loved ones was when they'd put them into the back of an ambulance and now they couldn't visit, or even call to find out how they were doing. They were totally reliant on us calling them, and when we did speak to them it was often from behind the main reception, a crowded and noisy area with constant interruptions.

So Tim and Anna, two consultant colleagues, set up the family liaison service. Led by Ian Needleman, a professor of dentistry, this was a team of volunteers from all around the hospital who manned phones twelve hours a day, seven days a week. Their home was an unused surgical seminar room with five phones and four computer terminals. They kept track of all the calls made, fielded calls from the families, passed on messages and ensured that each family received a medical update every day.

They also bought iPads and set up video calls. Sometimes, as with Jonathan and Megan, the video call was a two-way conversation, but at other times it was one way because the patient was sedated and ventilated. The iPad was clamped to a stand by the bed, and the relatives chatted away as if they were in the hospital sitting next to the patient. I don't think I would even have thought of it, and when I first heard the idea I was sceptical. Why would you want to stare at your poor husband or wife through an iPad when they were sedated on a ventilator and couldn't talk back to you? I was way off the mark. People normally visit sedated and ventilated loved ones, this was the closest we could offer, and the families grabbed the opportunity. The family liaison team managed it carefully. Recording settings were disabled, and warnings given, especially for young children, about what to expect, but after a few teething problems it became a huge success. Listening to a family, huddled around an iPad, chatting away to their loved one in a coma about what they'd been up to in lockdown was both moving and surprisingly life-affirming.

The restriction on visiting was and still is (visiting is still restricted, so we have kept a small family liaison team and the ability to video call in place) one of the most heartbreaking aspects of the Covid crisis. Speaking on the telephone to the loved one of a critically sick patient who is desperately trying to make sense of what is happening to their husband, wife, father or daughter feels wrong. I know it had to happen and perhaps it still does, but the psychological impact on patients and their families should not be underestimated. It makes a stay in ICU a very different experience for everyone.

Jonathan settled well on to the ventilator. His intubation was uneventful, and his oxygen levels manageable. I felt optimistic and called Megan back. Again she was calm and grateful and again the background noises in her home seemed so familiar. Perhaps that is why I was so desperate for him to recover. Or perhaps it was just my state of mind at the time. My adrenaline levels had dropped by the third week of April, and the grim reality of Covid was hitting home. I was seeing fewer patients skirt through ICU on CPAP and recover, because most of those were being managed upstairs on the HDRU. The ones we ventilated seemed to either go on and on being critically sick and unstable or nose-dive and die. Hardly any of them had recovered and come off the ventilator. I was increasingly anxious that we were doing something wrong and I was desperate for some good news.

On the day we intubated Jonathan, 17 April 2020, the UK national death toll for Covid positive patients reached 14,576. Ninety-nine-year-old Captain Tom completed 100 laps of his garden (raising more than £32 million), and the government announced another three weeks of lockdown. At UCH we were supposed to have been receiving a shipment of fifty new, state-of-the-art ICU ventilators from China. It was to be the end of our ventilator problems – with these new ones we'd have plenty to see us through the pandemic – but then on 12 April, a week before they were due to arrive they disappeared. The rumour was that Donald Trump had gazumped us.

It felt like a body blow at the time and deeply unjust. Every day we seemed to be on the verge of running out of decent ventilators, and we were constantly worried about the next batch of patients to come in through the door. Would we take a good ventilator off a patient who was doing badly to put it on to a new patient more likely to benefit, or perhaps put someone doing well on to an anaesthetic machine by the logic that they could probably get away with inferior equipment because they had more reserve? Was it OK to reduce someone's chances of surviving from 80 per cent to 70 per cent in order to improve someone else's chances from 30 per cent to 50 per cent? What if the first patient was forty years old and the second sixty? Did that make a difference? These were the ethical dilemmas we'd been dreading from the start, and it felt every day as if we were on the cusp of making some horrible choices. As ethics lead, perhaps I felt this even more keenly, but I didn't have any answers. These were complex philosophical questions. We could debate them for decades and come to no firm conclusion.

As it turned out, David, Rik, Geoff, Ramani and others were doing an extraordinary job of keeping just enough ventilators trickling into the hospital each day, and as the numbers started to plateau and the pressure for ventilators eased, the conversation at consultant meetings moved on. The question now was, how best to get all these patients off their ventilators?

Broadly there were two schools of thought, and I was firmly with the second. We'd already agreed that, once put to sleep, Covid patients should be kept deeply sedated and fully ventilated for the first few days to rest the lungs, minimize damage and allow the inflammation to improve. The hope was that over a week or so the blood markers would settle and the oxygen requirement come down, at which point we could lighten the sedation and allow the patients to start breathing. They'd still be receiving support from the ventilator with each breath, but gradually they'd do more and more of the work themselves and the ventilator less and less. Eventually after a few days they'd be doing the whole of each breath on their own, and we could disconnect them from the ventilator and take out the breathing tube.

The problem was that the Covid patients were not getting better after a week. Most were still inflamed and unstable not just after one week, but two and often three. Each time they seemed to be making progress, we'd lighten the sedation, start to get them breathing, their oxygen levels would plummet, and we were back to square one. Some of them had also progressed to a different phase. Their lungs were now getting stiffer, so delivering each breath required higher pressures. We hate delivering high pressures to the lungs because we know it causes damage, but without uncomfortably high pressure we couldn't adequately ventilate.

The first school of thought felt that we should exchange the oral breathing tube for a tracheostomy, lighten the sedation and push the patients forward, encouraging them to breathe for themselves, even if their lungs were stiff and their oxygen requirements high.

Tracheostomies (tubes through the neck into the trachea) are not only shorter and so easier to breathe through than tubes through the mouth, but also more comfortable, because they bypass the vocal cords. Having a breathing tube put through your vocal cords is more painful than having a surgical skin incision, so emerging from a prolonged induced coma with one still in place is distressing and disorientating. When people have been ventilated for more than ten days or so they usually need a tracheostomy as part of the weaning process – a stepping stone towards coming off the ventilator.

The thinking behind this strategy was that by inserting tracheostomies and encouraging the patients to breathe, they would need less sedatives, they'd suffer less delirium and muscle weakness, they'd wake up more quickly and so they should take less time to come off the ventilator. This is in line with modern ICU thinking. We always try to reduce sedation and make progress if we can, because the less time people spend on the ventilator the better, but with Covid patients it felt different. The course of their illness was more prolonged and complex and unpredictable than we were used to. Just when you thought you were getting somewhere, they'd spike a fever or throw off a blood clot or drop their oxygen levels or stop ventilating. We were still turning people on to their front as an emergency for catastrophically low oxygen levels three weeks into their illness. That was not normal.

The second school of thought, for which I was an advocate, was that we needed to be patient. For Covid patients we should wait, ride out the rocky course with them deeply asleep and us in control. Accept the slower recovery and the delirium, delay the tracheostomy and only try to make progress when they were clearly showing signs of being ready.

As one colleague put it, 'Note when you would normally start to wake them up, wait for forty-eight (or possibly seventy-two) hours, and if they still look good, go for it.'

The idea behind this strategy was that it would minimize damage to the lungs, maintain as much control as possible and avoid high-risk tracheostomies on unstable patients. We could put the tracheostomies in later if required, when the patients were more stable and the risks of the procedure lower. If they needed more sedation and took longer to wake up, so be it, they'd get there in the end. This approach would also reduce the chances of needing to prone people with tracheostomies, which, though possible, was not an attractive prospect.

As ever, there were strong opinions and no evidence, but this was a debate we never really resolved during the first surge.

Rik wanted to get on with the tracheostomies. Subsequently he described an overwhelming urge to do the next thing and keep moving forward. We'd prepared, we'd expanded, we'd CPAPed, we'd ventilated; now it was time to tracheostomize. So Rik, being Rik, got on with it.

He contacted the ENT surgeons and two of our most experienced intensivists (both groups insert tracheostomies, depending on the physical characteristics of the patient), and together they worked out an SOP. A day later Haydar received the first Covid tracheostomy, and it was a success: safely inserted with minimal risk to the staff. A few days after that, Rik added 'tracheostomies' as an agenda item to the daily SitRep meetings. The ICU consultants identified candidates before the meeting, the details were passed on to the 'trachey team', and up to four were inserted each day. It was impressive, but I still had misgivings.

People seemed to be obsessed with tracheostomies all of a sudden, as if moving the breathing tube to the neck was going to be some miracle cure for Covid, and the more we could put in the better. It felt wrong to me, as if we were rounding people up for tracheostomies. Not asking if anyone might benefit from one, but rather saying, 'If you can't give me a good reason not to, I'm putting one in, so we can turn down the sedation, get them breathing and move forward.'

There is always pressure to be doing something in ICU, and deciding to change nothing and sit on your hands can be the hardest position to take. It can feel timid or lacking in imagination and ideas, but I have come to the conclusion that 'masterful inactivity' is often the right course of action. Time, as we all know, is a great healer.

I didn't articulate this well at the time and I still don't know if I was right. Rik and other colleagues, with the help of the ENT surgeons, successfully sited more than forty tracheostomies in Covid patients, and many of them did very well. In preparation for another surge, we have debated the issue again and agreed to delay tracheostomies until the patients have been ventilated for two weeks at the earliest. I considered that a victory; others might call it a compromise.

This was a low point for me. The numbers were still not

falling, and lots of people had died. I was worried that we were slightly losing our way. There were hints from the data team that our outcome figures did not make pretty reading. At one point an email circulated around the consultants suggesting we might be looking at over 60 per cent mortality. This turned out to be the inverse of the truth, but it hit me hard. If the rumours about the outcomes from other hospitals were true, it implied we'd got this badly wrong.

I am usually fairly accepting of death. I do my best, but when the outlook is hopeless or the patient has had enough, I am pragmatic. Having said that, I am far from blasé about my own death. I am not religious, but I am anxious and the concept of oblivion is not one I find easy to accept, so I tend to rely on the fact that I don't know when death will happen to avoid ruminating on the subject. If I was given a date and time, I suspect I might spend half my life checking my watch and counting down the days. As a result, perhaps, when I am dealing with patients whose outlook is poor I tend to be at the 'keep going a bit longer' end of the spectrum, compared to my colleagues. Whilst many of them are rightly horrified by the pain and anguish that we put patients through on ICU for potentially small gains, I struggle more with the uncertainty of the outcome. I worry about the small chance that we might deny a patient meaningful life, and then about what denotes meaningful life, and finally how that varies from person to person. But I am not an outlier. I understand the limitations of what we can offer and I recognize the downsides of delaying inevitable death.

In the second half of April, though, I had had enough. I couldn't face more people dying. I wanted to keep everyone going, to rescue them all, however bleak it looked. It was a new disease, and we didn't know the future, so we should keep trying until their hearts actually stopped. I tell myself that this was because I wanted to give every patient every possible chance, and it was to a large extent, but I was also dealing with my own moral injury and if I am *completely* honest I was fretting about our outcomes. When this was all over, our mortality rates would be compared with other hospitals around London, the UK and the whole world. We were all treating one disease, so for once we could be compared. We were using different clinical strategies, and rumours were already circulating that certain hospitals were doing better than others.

I was also worried that we were at risk of slipping into a pandemic mindset. Rather than treat every patient as an individual, with a unique set of reasons to live, we might start to view them as a herd. There were so many patients and they were so sick that there was a danger in my mind we'd get too used to death and become too accepting. I was scared we might start viewing it as normal and inevitable. Our three wise people approach mitigated this. For a patient to be deemed hopeless there needed to be unanimity amongst the group, and on many occasions there wasn't, but even the three wise people system was fallible. If the majority opinion on the shop floor was that a case was hopeless then to push back was hard. 'Flogging' hopeless cases can be awful for staff, particularly the nurses who spend their whole day with the patient. It is easy for me to say keep going and then move on to the next patient, but for the nurse looking after the patient it can feel cruel, pointless and undignified. While I might be traumatized by the possibility of not persisting long enough with certain patients, other staff may be haunted by those to whom we'd denied a dignified death.

Alice is a good example of this. She is one of the most compassionate, hard-working and conscientious doctors I have ever met and she is deeply affected by the suffering of patients on the ICU. She has told me in the past that if she was on a ventilator and it didn't look good after a few days, she'd want us to stop. Other colleagues would not want to be ventilated on ICU at all.

They have seen how the physical and psychological insult debilitates patients, not just in the short term but often for years afterwards, and they do not feel it is worth it. For them personally, the ends do not justify the means. They are the minority, and I have slight doubts about whether they'd stick to this position when actually faced with the alternative, but I may be wrong. Perhaps they are just much more accepting of death than I am.

On 22 April I was on a night shift. Earlier that day I'd heard that a BBC team were coming to film a documentary on the unit to be presented by the Van Tulleken twins, and the news just compounded my despondency (not because of the Van Tullekens, I think they are great; for a period my children worshipped them, and for some reason Tish finds *Operation Ouch* very watchable). For years I'd bemoaned the lack of public understanding of ICU and I had even agreed before Covid to take part in a fly-on-the-wall documentary, but now this programme seemed just another reminder of the state of the world. Everything was Covid, it was all we were talking about, everything else was on hold, and there was no end in sight. By now 18,100 people had died with Covid in the UK, and Chris Whitty was describing the chances of finding an effective treatment or vaccine within the next calendar year as 'incredibly small'.

At the beginning I'd viewed the pandemic as a three-month process. The virus would come, it would be awful, and then it would go again, but now it seemed it was staying. We needed to stop dreaming of a post-Covid world and start working out ways to live with it. There was no guarantee of a vaccine, there is no HIV or SARS vaccine, and, even if they made one, there'd be another virus. We might be entering a new era of facemasks and social distancing. Things I took for granted, like travel, live entertainment and socializing, might never be the same. I was mourning normality. I'd complained so bitterly about Brexit and worried so much about climate change, but I'd never even considered this.

I was hoping this night shift might be quieter. The numbers were still high, but new admissions were down, and the patients were more established. Hopefully they'd be in a steady state, at least for my twelve hours in charge. As soon as I saw the dayshift consultants, though, I realized that I was kidding myself. They looked exhausted. As they talked through the patients, it became clear that they'd gone for the 'lighten sedation and get the patients breathing' strategy. Many patients now had tracheostomies, and most were initiating their own breaths on the ventilator. They were all still requiring a high amount of oxygen, but there was positivity in the room. It had been tiring, and there were lots of sick patients, but the day team felt that we were making progress.

There was one piece of unequivocally good news. Haydar, the man whom Rik, Mervyn and I had felt so pessimistic about in our three wise people session three weeks previously, had been discharged to the ward. After six weeks on ICU, kidney failure, pressure sores, blood clots, respiratory failure and our first Covid tracheostomy, he'd got better. He still had problems, the pressure sore on his cheek from lying on his front was yet to heal, and he was as weak as a kitten, but his vital organs were working. He no longer needed machines and he'd escaped from ICU. He was the first long-term sick patient to get better, and it felt like a major triumph.

Then Shaima joined us.

Shaima is an obstetric anaesthetist who'd volunteered to move over to ICU. She is a consummate professional, but she wears it lightly and usually looks serene and mildly amused. That night she looked defeated.

'Are you OK?' I asked

'No, not really,' she replied. 'Good luck and . . . sorry.'

'Where have you—?'

'Bay 4. It's . . . awful. I've tried, but they're just so . . . sick, well three out of four.'

Shaima spent six months as a registrar in Ethiopa working for VSO. While out there she set up an ICU, the first in that region, covering a population of eight million people. It was a harrowing experience, she told me, during which she felt stretched and out of control, almost constantly. She left more grateful than ever for the NHS, but during Covid, for the first time since Ethiopia, she had that feeling again – 'as if I needed to divide myself in three and be with all the patients all the time'.

The people Shaima was talking about were established patients who now had a combination of respiratory problems. Their lungs were still inflamed, so difficult to get oxygen in through, but also stiff and so difficult to ventilate adequately to clear carbon dioxide. Many of them also had clots in the blood vessels to the lungs, making both oxygen and carbon dioxide more difficult to handle.

These problems are not unique to Covid, but what did seem more prevalent was the stark choice to be made. You could either deeply sedate the patients, fully control the ventilation and optimize the oxygen or lighten the sedation to allow the patients to breathe up and clear more carbon dioxide. It was one or the other, you couldn't have both. Inevitably there was no evidence, lots of theory and different opinions about the best option to take. I think if you were on the side of watching and waiting generally for Covid patients you naturally favoured the former, whereas if you were keen to push forward and get them breathing early, your inclination was to go for the latter. The issues were all tangled together, and again, although I like to think I reacted to the individual patient in front of me and tailored my plan to their needs, the truth was that I just preferred to control the ventilation.

My colleagues from the day shift, however, had gone for the latter. As I walked round the patients that night, I was struck by how many of them were tugging away at their ventilators, their heads pulling to the side for each breath. It made me feel uneasy. They were sedated so were unaware, but they *looked* uncomfortable, and while the carbon dioxide was under control, their oxygen requirements were rising.

Meddling with the clinical plans from the day, when you are only there for a night shift, should not be done lightly. ICU care relies on a consistent approach, and chopping and changing on a whim only hinders progress. When registrars change my plans without good reason I feel irritated and undermined and often become defensive, but that night I was torn. My pet teaching topic is ventilation, and I'd convinced myself that I was right. This was my thing, and I felt uncomfortable looking at all these patients who seemed to be struggling away, so in the end I went around changing things. I could justify it – their oxygen levels were deteriorating – but I knew it wasn't just that. A part of me was just determined to be right.

Each time I deepened the sedation, paralysed and took over the ventilation, the transition was nerve-racking. The oxygen levels dive-bombed initially, teetered perilously close to disaster, and then only ever so slowly climbed back up again. Each patient recovered to a new steady state, but if I am honest, not an objectively better one. They looked more peaceful and comfortable and some had better oxygen levels, but the carbon dioxide levels were worse. I could convince myself I'd made some gains, but I'd have struggled to convince anyone else. Shaima's three 'sickies' and one other patient were still *in extremis*. The only option left was to turn them on to their fronts.

Juan, a previously fit Filipino nurse who worked in elderly care and looked much younger than his sixty-one years, had been a patient on the unit for just over a week. Two days previously the team had sited a tracheostomy, only four days after putting him on a ventilator. Now he was on 100 per cent oxygen, but still his blood oxygen levels were falling. His lungs had deteriorated dramatically, he was highly inflamed and he needed to be turned on to his front, but it would have been so much easier if the tube was still through his mouth. I found myself mumbling angrily into my FFP3 mask.

'Why the hell have you put a trachey in after four days? He's got weeks of ventilation ahead of him. What's the upside? He might not need one at all. What is this bloody obsession?'

This was grossly unfair and far more a reflection of my state of mind than reality, but I was agitated as I assembled a team, put four pillows under Juan's chest and turned him on to his front. He coped well with the turn, and his oxygen levels improved, but his tracheostomy was now difficult to access, so suctioning secretions from his chest was awkward. If the tube had become displaced that night, with him on his front, it might well have been fatal and it would have been my problem, not the person who'd decided to put it in in the first place.

Again, these complaints are not fair. The tracheostomy had been inserted in good faith, but I was getting fractious. Many of us were. We'd had enough, and still, despite being on their fronts, three of the four patients were in imminent danger. So I tried something new.

Occasionally we put 5-litre bags of fluid on patients' chests. The idea is that the weight redistributes ventilation within the lungs and so improves oxygen levels. We sometimes try it when proning is not possible, as the effect is thought to be similar, but these three patients were already on their fronts – so what about putting the 5-litre bag of fluid on their backs? I'd never seen it, or even heard of it, but I was exhausted and out of ideas and maybe I'd had a moment of genius. People might talk about it for years to come, the 'Down Manoeuvre'. I got some funny looks from the nurses and trainees as I carefully balanced the bags in the optimum position between the shoulder blades, but I was the boss, so they didn't stop me. If anything, it seemed to help slightly, so I left the bags in place, patted myself on the back and set off for the Pods.

Three of the Pod patients that night had lungs as stiff as boards and carbon dioxide levels off the scale. They were all fully ventilated via tracheostomies, so I spent between 5 a.m. and 7 a.m. oscillating between their three beds. For two hours I fiddled with their ventilators, my sole aim being to reduce the carbon dioxide levels of three men in their early fifties. It was slow and painstaking, trial and error. With one tweak I'd make a small gain and with the next go back to where I'd started, but gradually the carbon dioxides crept down – not to normal levels, just down to three times higher than normality.

Eventually, having finally admitted I'd done all I could, I pulled off my PPE and shuffled back to the office for something to drink. As I sipped my pallid NHS tea, I thought through the 'Down Manoeuvre' and quickly realized that it made no physiological sense. It was harmless, but essentially I was fighting myself, so I slipped into a fresh set of PPE, nipped back into the bays and took all the fluid off the patients' backs before the day shift returned. It would be our little night-shift secret.

This period was frustrating and dispiriting for all of us, but the ICU nurses were having the worst of it.

They were still at full stretch, one nurse to four or five patients, and they couldn't deliver the level of care they were used to. Sedated ICU patients are helpless. They can't move, they can't cough, they can't swallow, they can't blink and they can't ask for or refuse any treatment. They can't tell someone who's approaching them without washing their hands to bugger off and they can't scream when they are in pain. They are completely reliant on their nurse. If they are left without being turned for a few hours they develop the first signs of pressure sores; a few more hours and the skin has broken down. A lack of eye lubrication results in abrasions, without mouth care they are at risk of pneumonia, and a drug error can be catastrophic. As well as running all the fancy machines, the ICU nurses look after all these vital functions. They are fastidious about repositioning their patients every two hours, they double-check every drug dose, question the prescriptions that don't make sense and assess the risks constantly.

Elaine had established an ethos of excellence at UCH, and the nurses were rightly proud of their record. They had seen the benefits. Pressure sores were almost unheard of, drug errors minimal, and hospital-acquired infections a rarity. These are the things that make a tangible difference to both the experience and the outcomes of ICU patients, and for the last five years the feedback from relatives and patients had reflected that.

But over the last few weeks, pressure sores were creeping back in. The eyes of proned patients looked swollen and bloodshot, and in full PPE infection control was almost impossible. The nurses were doing everything they could to keep their patients safe, but they were overwhelmed. They couldn't physically do what they wanted to for every patient, so they felt as if they were causing harm. They were also finding it harder to connect emotionally with the people in their care. There were no relatives by the bedside to humanize the patients, who were often lying face down for the whole shift. Some nurses telephoned the families and asked for personal information to help them build a relationship, but others found that too upsetting. This was no longer ICU nursing as they knew it, and there was also the ever-present anxiety about their own health. They looked after five colleagues on UCH ICU through the pandemic.

Elaine takes every pressure sore personally. She investigates, supports the staff involved, looks at what can be improved and institutes the necessary changes, but Covid put a stop to all that. For Elaine it was a double hit. This was harmful to the patients and deeply distressing for her nurses. Every day another member of staff arrived in her office in floods of tears. Some were exhausted, some frightened, and many were just desperate to get back to delivering the highest standards of ICU care, but Elaine was as helpless as everyone else. There were no more ICU nurses.

Alice was the first consultant to realize just how bad it was for the nurses. We all knew it was tough, and I'd had my moment of enlightenment with Julie, but we had our own problems. We were the ones making the difficult decisions, bearing the weight of responsibility and trying to work out how best to treat this terrible disease. What we weren't doing, however, was running all day (in full PPE) struggling just to deliver decent ICU patient care. It was too easy in the pandemic to be self-obsessed, to think only of what a tough time you were having and to ignore the impact on those around you.

But Alice noticed and she decided the answer was to marshal the helpers. There were hundreds of them by now: redeployed nurses, medical students, surgeons, dentists – each morning the ICU was packed with people, so Alice gave them jobs. She organized them into rotas on shifts (including nights) and allocated them specific tasks, with the sole aim of allowing the nurses to deliver the best possible care. And it worked. The nurses started to feel more in control and when, at three o'clock one morning, I asked the whereabouts of more pillowcases, it was a vascular surgeon who showed me. He'd been working night shifts doing turns, washes, mouth and eye care and taking blood samples and knew exactly where the linen was kept.

And then Rik suggested we change our language. Rather

than ask, 'Could you do so and so?' we'd ask, 'Could you show me how to do so and so?' It was a small change, but such an important shift of mindset.

By the time I got to my run of day shifts at the end of April, we had a new problem with tracheostomies: they were leaking. About an inch from the tip of both tracheostomy and endotracheal tubes there is a cuff. Once in position, the cuff is inflated and forms a seal within the trachea to prevent the leak of air upwards, and vomit or anything else downwards. When tracheostomies do not sit well within the trachea, the cuff can fail to form a seal, meaning that with each breath air gurgles out through the mouth. The short-term solution is to reposition the tracheostomy tube and inflate the cuff with more air, but this is rarely more than a temporary fix. High pressure in the cuff causes damage to the tracheal wall, and repositioning doesn't work for long. The only definitive answer is to exchange the tube for a bigger or longer one.

The tracheostomies in Covid patients were leaking a lot. The virus seemed to damage the tracheal architecture of some patients, leaving it floppy and dilated.

Eli was a previously healthy, slim South African man in his early fifties. He had been ventilated since 27 March and then 'tracheyed' three days previously, but subsequently his ventilation had deteriorated. His oxygen requirements were going up, his lungs getting stiffer, and for the last twenty-four hours both problems had been compounded by a big leak of air around the tracheostomy cuff. By the time I took over his care, nearly a third of each breath was heading straight up out of the mouth rather than down to the lungs. Not only did that mean that he was receiving inadequate ventilation, it also meant that the background pressure delivered to his lungs was reduced, which in turn allowed airspaces to collapse each breath, reducing his oxygen levels and perpetuating the inflammation. I needed to change his tracheostomy.

Replacing an established tracheostomy is usually simple and takes less than twenty seconds, but Eli was on 100 per cent oxygen with blood oxygen sats of 88 per cent. Within seconds of being disconnected from the ventilator he'd be in trouble, and this was a fresh trachey, sited by surgeons just three days previously, so there was no established track for the new tube to follow. It could all go wrong very quickly, but it had to be done, so I called the ENT surgeons and we gathered our equipment and worked out our backup plans. Before starting, the ENT surgeon had a look down the tracheostomy with a fibre-optic scope and discovered that the trachea was indeed dilated and floppy.

'Very interesting,' he mused. But I was far more interested in the fact that I couldn't get Eli's oxygen sats above 85 per cent now and was starting to feel out of control.

'OK, now or never, I think,' I said.

'Sure?'

'Yup . . . yup, go for it.'

Within twenty seconds he'd slipped a suction catheter down through the tracheostomy, pulled out the old tube, leaving the catheter behind, and then railroaded a new longer tracheostomy back down over the catheter. I then inflated the cuff and began to ventilate the lungs with a bag. There was no leak, and the chest was rising. It couldn't have been smoother, and I let out a sigh of relief as I secured the new tracheostomy in position and connected it to the ventilator. Before leaving, the ENT surgeon had one last look down the tube with the fibre-optic scope and confirmed that it was well positioned. Job done.

'Great,' I said, 'thank you. I'll just get him settled, and then shall we do the other one in bay 3, say half an hour?'

We had an identical problem in the same bed of the next-door bay.

'See you there.'

As the ENT team left, I looked up at the monitor. Eli's oxygen sats were 79 per cent. In normal times that would have got my adrenaline pumping, but I was getting used to it. He had Covid, 79 per cent was run of the mill, it would pick up.

'Could someone call for an x-ray,' I asked, 'just to be sure.'

'Just doing it,' replied one of the SHOs, so I turned back to Eli.

His saturations were not picking up. Now they were 75 per cent.

'Bloody hell,' I mumbled gearing up for a protracted battle to get Eli properly oxygenated. Turning him on his front would not be ideal with a brand-new trachey and certainly not before a chest x-ray, so I needed to try everything else first. I fiddled with the ventilator settings, reparalysed him, leaned him to one side then the other, suctioned the lungs for secretions, bolstered the blood pressure and sat him up, but nothing seemed to make the slightest difference. If anything, things were getting worse.

His oxygen levels were now 72 per cent, and his heart rate was rising. Rik popped in to give a second opinion, had a look at everything I'd looked at and concurred with my thoughts. The sats briefly lifted to 80 per cent, so, reassured that this was no more than nasty Covid, he went on his way, but something wasn't right. Twenty minutes later the chest x-ray team had still not materialized, and the sats were now in the 60s, so I asked the SHO to phone them again and called Dave Brealey in to have a look. I noticed that his left lung was not expanding as well as his right but I couldn't listen for breath sounds, because we weren't using stethoscopes. I assumed it was due to a plug of phlegm blocking one of the main airways to the left side and so Dave tried some physiotherapy (shaking of the chest to free up secretions) to shift it, but to no avail. By the time the x-ray finally arrived, Eli's oxygen sats were 60, his pulse up to 140, and his blood pressure dropping fast. The radiographer slipped the x-ray plate behind Eli's back, and we all retreated. I glanced up at the monitor. He was in danger of going into cardiac arrest, so as Dave went back to check the image on the x-ray machine, I grabbed some adrenaline from the crash trolley.

And then Dave bolted for the door.

'CHEST DRAIN SET NOW!' he shouted into the corridor.

'Shit. No!'

'Yup, tension pneumothorax.'

I grabbed the biggest cannula I could find and plunged it through the front of Eli's chest. As I pulled the needle back out of the sheath, I listened for the hiss of air, but I couldn't hear anything through my PPE so I got a second cannula and pushed it in alongside the first and then followed that with a third. I still couldn't hear any air coming out, but the oxygen saturation and blood pressure started to creep in the right direction. Within a couple of minutes Dave was back by the bed space with a scalpel, chest drain, tubing and underwater seal. Two minutes after that, he made an incision in Eli's side, pushed apart the tissues with his finger until he was between two ribs and through the chest wall into the space around the lung and inserted a 30-cm plastic tube (the diameter of penne pasta). He then connected that tube to a second, longer piece of tubing and pushed the end of that into a bottle half filled with water. We watched with relief as air bubbled out through the water with each breath.

The chest x-ray of a tension pneumothorax is the one you should never see. Pneumothorax means air in the space between the lung and the chest wall, the pleural space. The air gets there by leaking out of damaged airways or lung tissue. Often, particularly when the patient is ventilated, a one-way ball valve effect occurs, meaning the air passes into the pleural space during inspiration but cannot escape during expiration. The expanding volume of gas in the pleural space pushes away the lung and eventually the heart. It is then called a tension pneumothorax and can eventually, if left unchecked, lead to cardiac arrest. The treatment is to drain the air and allow the lung to re-expand, initially with a cannula and then more formally with a drain, as we did – in the end. But the diagnosis should be clinical – reduced breath sounds and chest movement on one side, hyper-resonance to percussion (the tapping of one finger over another on the chest wall) and trachea pushed over to the other side. It should be identified and treated without the need of an x-ray, it's classic page one emergency medicine, but I'd missed it, with almost fatal consequences.

I missed it for two reasons. The first was that I didn't think of it. Eli had no reason to develop a tension pneumothorax at that moment, I'd never seen or heard of one following a simple change of tracheostomy, and we'd not forced particularly high pressure into his lungs. In addition, he had plenty of other reasons to have low oxygen levels. I'd made the assumption this was just another case of awful Covid and failed to pause and think laterally.

The second reason I missed it was that I didn't, and perhaps couldn't, examine him properly. I couldn't listen to his chest, because we were not using stethoscopes, and I couldn't usefully percuss it, because I was wearing three pairs of gloves.

On 30 April, Tricia, the head of nursing from GOSH whom Max and Dan had intubated three weeks previously and who had accepted her situation with such stoicism and dignity, reached the end of the line. Her lungs were still getting worse, her kidneys had failed, and her heart was requiring more and more support. There was nowhere else to go. We had turned her on to her front, we had tried fully ventilating her and we had tried letting her breathe (she'd always been far too sick for a tracheostomy). We'd tried anticoagulation, antibiotics, steroids, plasma exchange, kidney support and different regimes for the heart, but nothing had changed her trajectory. She was dying but she was under my care again, and I was struggling to accept it. Like everyone else, I'd run out of options, but I couldn't let go. There must be something more we could do. I talked to several colleagues, but the conversations just confirmed what deep down I already knew, so I called in her family.

During the hour and a half it took for Tricia's family to travel up from Broadstairs, I started to dread the conversation. What would I say? Would they be angry? Would they be medical and question our decisions and treatment? She was only sixty, a few weeks before she'd been fine, the head of nursing for haematology and oncology at GOSH.

By the time I walked into the relatives' room I was anxious and paranoid, already second-guessing what they might ask. There were six or seven of them in the room, including her husband, twenty-year-old daughter Emily and seventeen-year-old son Luke. They looked shattered, but they smiled at me warmly as I perched on my customary bin. I introduced myself and carefully explained the situation, and they listened quietly and nodded. I said that Tricia was still on full organ support, but nevertheless deteriorating and that if things continued on this course she was unlikely to survive the night. When I'd finished, I paused and waited for their questions, but there weren't any, so I added that we'd of course make sure that she didn't suffer and offered them a final visit to the bedside. Again they nodded and silently wrapped comforting arms around each other.

Eventually her husband looked up.

'We understand,' he said, 'you've done all you can, but this is just what it is. We know. Thank you.'

There was no anger, no hostility and no bitterness. They were all desperately sad to be losing their beloved Tricia, it was painful, unfair and heartbreaking, but if it was time to let go then that is what they would do. I glanced around the room one more time to check that there were no more questions, but they were not looking for anything more from me. They were each individually tying to comprehend and come to terms with their loss, and for that they needed each other, their family.

I walked out of the hospital that night feeling wretched, a part of me still hoping that by some miracle Tricia might turn the corner and pull through. I felt helpless and hopeless and guilty. I couldn't get all the 'what ifs' out of my head.

'What if we'd intubated her earlier?'

'What if we'd tried a different experimental drug? Or a different dose of steroids? Or different antibiotics? Or if we'd kept her more deeply sedated, or less deeply sedated?'

Each of these things might have made things a bit better, or worse, but far more likely would have made no difference.

There is nothing to suggest we did anything wrong with the care of Tricia, but at the time I was deeply unsure. It was as if the ICU carpet had been pulled from under me. I'd started to doubt my knowledge, my decisions and my judgement – and not just mine, everyone else's as well. I was doing my best, I thought, but it didn't seem to be enough. The pandemic had stabilized, but it wasn't going away. We were still bringing in more patients, and we didn't seem to be making them better. Tricia was just another in a series of patients who'd gradually deteriorated to the point of no return. How many more of the sixty or so still on the unit would end up going the same way?

To have tripled the size of our ICU was an enormous achievement, but at the end of April I was starting to wonder if it had all been worthwhile. If we were just delaying the inevitable, what was the point? There was still no evidence that any specific intervention made a difference, the vaccine seemed a million years away, and normality was rapidly becoming a distant memory. I couldn't see a way out of this. My colleagues were exhausted and fed up, the economy was in freefall and the backlog of 'normal medicine' – cancer, heart disease and diabetes – was unimaginable. The hidden costs to the health of the country would be enormous.

I pushed open my front door and grunted a vague 'hey' into the hallway.

'Dad, DAD!' Tom was bounding down the stairs towards me. 'Hi, come and look at the new computer. It's amazing. Mum's ordered me a mouse!'

Tom leaped from the bottom step into my arms and hugged me.

'Pleasure.' I replied. 'For homework too, though, remember.'

'Da-ad! Don't ruin it.'

With Tom still in my arms I looked up to see Edie leaning nonchalantly against the banisters, her phone, as ever, in her hand.

' 'Sup, Dad?' she asked, then smiled and joined in the hug.

'Hi, Edie, you OK?'

'Dad, can we go to the shop? I've got my own money.'

'The shop's shut, Edes, but I nicked a packet of digestives from work.'

'You stole them?'

'No. Well . . . I'll replace them, promise.'

The next day I telephoned my colleague, Tim, who'd been on overnight. Tricia had died at 5 a.m., he told me, sleeping peacefully and her family had asked that he pass on their thanks to all the people who'd looked after her.

8. Recovery

1 May 2020

On the morning Tricia died I was working in a local private hospital. I cover their nine-bedded, predominantly surgical, ICU three days a month in normal times (outside of my NHS time), but for the first few weeks of Covid it had all but shut down. Like the NHS, they'd stopped elective surgery and minimized admissions to reduce the risk of spreading Covid through the hospital.

Then, in early April, the private hospital (along with others) signed a contract with the NHS, and within a week NHS patients were having major cancer surgery in the private sector. The ICU where I work expanded from nine to sixteen beds, and the first weekend in May was my weekend on.

When I arrived at the hospital I was immediately struck by how calm and quiet it was. I showed my ID badge through the glass front door, which then slid silently aside, allowing me to bow my head and have my temperature checked. Having passed that test, I proceeded to the sink to wash my hands and received a crisp, fresh mask. Screened, cleaned and masked, I then rode an empty lift to the fourth floor, where I helped myself to a latte from the coffee room before joining the two junior doctors in the office to hear about the patients.

As they described the third well patient in a row, who was sitting out of bed after a colon resection, my mind wandered back to UCH and all the patients who were sedated, ventilated and clinging to life. I felt guilty, but also relieved to have a moment of respite.

We wore full PPE to see the patients. There was one small donning station in the middle of the unit with neat piles of hats, masks, gloves and gowns, but I wasn't quite sure if the PPE was to protect us or them. The patients had all isolated for two weeks and been scrupulously screened for Covid before coming in, whereas I'd just come from Covid-ridden UCH ICU, but either way PPE had become second nature by now, and the ward round was a pleasure. These NHS patients were awake and delighted to have had their cancers removed. They had diseases that I understood and were on established pathways, so I soon settled into the routine of surgical ICU.

'Is your pain under control? Have you been out of bed? Have you passed wind? Do you feel sick? What are you watching on TV?'

In five to seven days' time they'd go home and in three months they'd have fully recovered. It was a relief to chat calmly to patients, examine them *with a stethoscope* and send them on their way. By lunchtime I'd seen all twelve patients and set up plans.

Through the pandemic 600 major cancer operations were performed on NHS patients from North Central and North East London alone in private hospitals.

I walked back to UCH with a spring in my step.

There were 631 Covid deaths reported on 1 May in the UK, down from a peak of 1,172 in mid April. The total number was over 30,000, but at UCH we admitted no new Covid patients to ICU that day for the first time in more than six weeks. It wasn't over: we were still bursting with patients and we'd admit many more over the subsequent weeks, but Rik had decided it was time for us to reflect on what we had achieved so far, so he called us to a meeting. At 2 p.m., forty of us gathered in the UCH education centre.

We spread across the flat, low-ceilinged lecture theatre at individual chair-desks, like socially distanced GCSE candidates in a sports hall. All the big guns were there: the chief executive, the medical directors and several other people in suits, so important that I didn't even recognize them. The idea was that we'd hear five-minute presentations from each clinical group involved in the pandemic response – what they'd done, what they'd learned and what they'd do differently next time.

My remit was to speak about Ethics. By now, Baroness Julia Neuberger had chaired several meetings of the Clinical Ethics Advisory Group (the first on Good Friday), and we had produced local guidance on decision-making and ethical principles in a pandemic. We had also put plans in place to audit the quality of the decisions we made through the Covid crisis. To learn and improve we needed to examine both how we had made decisions and what we had decided in terms of withhold and withdrawal of treatments. That way we could have an honest discussion about whether we'd do anything differently next time. Officially the ethical framework had never shifted. There had been a lot of argument about a move from fairness to benefit, but as far as the government was concerned we had never hit the limits of resource, so no change was required. On one level I couldn't argue with that, but it didn't tell the whole story of the reality on the shop floor. We may never quite have run out of equipment nationally, but the quality varied, we did run out of trained staff, and for periods some hospitals were completely overwhelmed. Nevertheless, we needed to examine what we had done so that we could learn and set up systems to minimize the chances of repeating any mistakes.

I delivered a very brief talk to that effect and then sat down to listen to twenty other presentations.

There was little I didn't already know, but it was extraordinary to have it all laid out again. The speed and scale of the hospital's transformation was breathtaking. Two new ICUs had been set up, and we'd treated over 190 critically sick Covid patients. Nine ICU physiotherapists had become forty-nine, a brand-new transfer team had transported nearly fifty ICU patients into UCH, and the tactical team had held three meetings a day to redistribute patients and equipment, not just across the trust, but around the whole of North London. Almost everyone in the hospital was working a new rota, with over 100 staff arriving on ICU alone every shift. Family communication was now all remote, new guidelines were being written and updated every day, fifty anaesthetists had become intensivists whilst others were now facilitating cancer surgery elsewhere, a whole floor of the hospital was newly devoted to stock, swathes of the Trust IT system had been reconfigured, radiologists had formed lines teams, medical students proning teams and surgeons were working as nursing assistants. The national hospital for neurology and neurosurgery had become a Covid hospital, staff wellbeing clinics were up and running and we were participating in six Covid clinical trials. There was no new scientific evidence yet, but many lessons had already been learned, and people were tentatively planning for the future.

Rik is a brilliant man, but he's still got a lot to learn about chairing a meeting. There was too much on the agenda and with only five minutes per talk inevitably everyone overran (basic, level-one chairing), so by the time our medical director stood up, nearly three hours after me, to talk about future green, blue and amber patient pathways in a gold, silver and bronze hierarchy, I had reached the end of my attention span and slipped out the back to do my afternoon ward round. The 'post-Covid' plans were bound to change; I'd catch up later.

On 4 May (a bank holiday, although no one noticed) Fergus Walsh and his cameraman Adam Walker returned to UCH. It had been a month since their original BBC piece, and the idea was to see how things had progressed and to gauge how we felt about the future. Unfortunately, in my case the answer to the second question was 'not good'. A week later, it would have been a slightly different story, but on 4 May I was still gloomy. I was not on for the ICU, but I'd caught up with the patients on the main unit, who were still very sick, and my brief excursion into the private sector had only served to remind me of how life used to be.

Other worries too were creeping into my head. Everyone's enthusiasm for home schooling was wearing thin (or thinner), and there was no prospect of it ending before September. Tom and Edie were meant to be attempting the eleven-plus at Christmas, and their preparation seemed to me haphazard despite our best efforts. From the family Zoom calls it was apparent that my mother's dementia was progressing rapidly, and although my father and brother were doing a fantastic job of looking after her, I had no idea of when I'd next be able to visit and whether by then she'd even recognize me.

I think Fergus was looking for the green shoots of recovery in this second interview, and in retrospect I wish I had given him some, but at the time I couldn't find it in me to be anything but downbeat. After a strange, lingering long shot during which I stared down the lens doing my best Nick Cave impersonation, I essentially told him that the disease was 'brutal, and going nowhere' and that I was still 'shell-shocked by the whole experience'. I thought I was just neutrally and accurately reporting the situation in our hospital, but, looking back at the tape, I think I was still traumatized by the Tricias and Adams I'd looked after. I could see that lockdown had worked and that the numbers were falling, but we still had fifty critically ill Covid patients, and I was terrified that they might all die.

After my interview of doom and gloom it was Elaine's turn,

and if anything she was even more negative. She spoke about the impact on her staff and described being 'haunted by images of rows of patients lying faceless on their fronts'. So it wasn't just me, then.

We then repeated the ward round of a month previously, back in the Pods. It started badly, when I discovered that two of the patients whose carbon dioxides I'd struggled with on my last night shift had passed away. They were young men my age, and although I'd known they were in trouble, it was a shock to hear that they'd both died. There was, however, some good news.

Andrew was a forty-five-year-old IT manager. He'd got married in 2019 in a small ceremony in Gibraltar and planned to have a proper celebration in Sorrento in August 2020, but in the last week of March he'd caught Covid. He was fit apart from some mild asthma, but the virus had hit him hard, and on 6 April he came into UCH. A CT scan the next day revealed both inflammation and blood clots in his lungs, and he was given oxygen and blood thinners. A day later he was started on CPAP on the HDRU.

I first met him five days after that. I'd gone up to HDRU to decide whether he should come down to ICU and discovered him sitting out in his chair, curled forward over his tray table (self-proning). He had a CPAP mask strapped tight to his face and looked exhausted, but when I suggested he come down to ICU for closer monitoring, he shook his head.

'I'm OK,' he reassured me, 'I'd rather stay here.'

I interpreted his polite refusal as stoicism, but he told me later that he viewed going to ICU as 'crossing a threshold', highlighting that he was deteriorating and giving up on the trial treatments he'd recently started. He was well aware of the consequences if he deteriorated and wrote this message on his phone to a close friend: 'If my lungs give way first and stop taking CPAP, then I have to be ventilated. A lot of folk don't wake up from the ventilator.'

Andrew's trial treatments were a five-day course of plasma exchange and an anti-viral, and he was very hopeful that one or both might turn things around.

Blood is made up of cells (red blood cells, white blood cells and platelets) and plasma (everything else). In plasma exchange blood flows out of the body to be separated into cells and plasma. The plasma is then discarded while the cells are combined with fresh plasma from healthy blood donors and returned to the patient. One treatment takes about two hours and it is a well-established and effective therapy for many conditions, particularly those in which patients have developed antibodies against themselves. We offer plasma exchange twenty-four hours a day at UCH as an emergency life-saving treatment for a condition called Thrombotic Thrombocytopaenic Purpura. We didn't know if it would work in Covid, but the logic was that it would remove some of the drivers of inflammation. Other centres would try a modification of this and return 'hyperimmune' plasma from donors who'd already had Covid and developed antibodies. That strategy aimed to transfer the immunity of ex-patients to current patients.

After every 'exchange' Andrew felt better for a few hours. His temperature and heart rate settled, and his breathing eased, but by later each day he was almost back to where he'd started. For the moment, however, he and the medical team felt that he was coping, so I left him where he was.

A day later he was down on ICU, and a day or two after that, asleep, ventilated, on 100 per cent oxygen and turned on to his front.

Three weeks after that, however, when I went round with the BBC, he was showing signs of improvement. His oxygen requirements were reducing, and his lungs, though still inflamed, were expanding nicely. He'd undergone a second, five-day course of plasma exchange and two cycles of antibiotics and spent many days on his front, but at last he seemed to be getting better.

Many patients were still struggling, but there was one memorable moment with the BBC which, in retrospect, was probably a turning point for me. It was when we took them to see Thanasis. Thanasis was the big Greek man whom Paavan and I had struggled with for an hour after his intubation a month previously. The man we had turned on to his front as an emergency, but only made things worse, so then turned back again immediately. For the next week he'd been touch and go, but he'd clung on and then gradually clawed his way forward. On 19 April the ENT surgeons had inserted a tracheostomy, and after that we'd weaned down his sedation. Initially he was delirious, and I worried that the period of low oxygen had damaged his brain permanently, but after two more weeks his mind cleared. Soon after that he was well enough to breathe without the ventilator, and his tracheostomy was removed.

When Fergus, Adam and I entered the bay, Thanasis was on the phone. He was engrossed in a conversation, speaking animatedly in Greek to his wife, so we waited patiently at the end of his bed; three men in full PPE, one carrying a microphone on an extension, one with a BBC camera and me. Thanasis seemed not to notice us, and we were close to giving up when suddenly he looked up, and a huge smile spread across his face.

'BBC?' he shouted, throwing his phone (and so presumably his wife) into the bed clothes.

'Yes,' Fergus replied, as Adam turned his camera to face Thanasis. 'Sorry to interrupt, I was wondering . . .'

'Hello, LONDON!!' Thanasis bellowed, both arms in the air giving the camera a double thumbs-up.

'Hello, Thanasis. I was wondering if you'd mind if we asked—'

'HELLO, GREAT BRITAIN! HELLO, GREECE! I LOVE YOU.'

Even Fergus couldn't suppress a smile.

Thanasis went on to give the BBC a twenty-minute interview (much of which was in Greek, I believe), and I walked out of that bay grinning for the first time in weeks.

It turned out that Thanasis was the first of many. This was not just a turning point for me: the first week of May was when the whole ICU began to move forward. The influx of patients slowed to a trickle, and some who'd been with us almost since the beginning were starting to get better.

A great example was Driton, an athletic forty-four-year-old Kosovan plasterer who arrived back from the Royal Brompton Hospital on 4 May. We had admitted him to UCH three weeks previously with severe Covid and quickly needed to intubate and ventilate, but a CT scan of his chest the next day threw up a surprise. As well as the lung inflammation and blood clots we'd expected there was a pocket of air around his heart. This air must have leaked from a small perforation in his airways or lungs, and although it wasn't causing problems at that moment, if allowed to get bigger, it would. Just as the air that leaked from Eli's lung had compressed it, so this air might go on to compress Driton's heart. The difference was that the air around Driton's heart was not easily drainable. The obvious way to stop it expanding was to stop blowing air into the lungs, i.e. to stop ventilating him, but we could only do that if we found an alternative way to get the oxygen into his bloodstream and the carbon dioxide out.

That was where the Royal Brompton Hospital came in. They could offer him ExtraCorporeal Membrane Oxygenation (ECMO). ECMO involves pumping the blood out of a patient, oxygenating it, removing the carbon dioxide and returning it – essentially doing the work of the lungs and heart for them. It is delivered in a few specialist centres around the UK and is complex, expensive and carries serious risks, but for the right patient it can be life-saving. I'd felt that Driton was a perfect candidate for ECMO, the team at the Brompton agreed, and within two hours they had dispatched a team to pick him up. For the next sixteen days he was attached to an ECMO machine and so barely needed ventilation. Without air being forced in and out of the lungs, the tissues healed, and after a couple of weeks, both the leak and the lung inflammation had settled. By the time he came back to us he was a different man. He was profoundly weak, so needed two more weeks on the ventilator recuperating, but he never looked back.

And each day there were more encouraging signs. The strange thing was that, having been at death's door for weeks, once these patients began to get better they did so remarkably quickly. They should have taken weeks, months even, to come off the ventilator; they'd had severely inflamed and scarred lungs, deep, prolonged sedation and paralysis, kidney failure, periods with low oxygen and high-dose steroids. Each one of these factors makes weaning from a ventilator more difficult. The paralysis and steroids weaken the muscles, the sedatives, kidney failure and low oxygen addle the brain, and the inflamed and scarred lungs speak for themselves, but many of these patients came off their ventilators in days. It was as if a switch had been thrown, and it was time to get better. Even I was starting to feel optimistic.

On 8 May I sat down for a three wise people discussion with Alice and Mike (another ICU consultant, and medical director at the FA, who should have been away preparing for Euro 2020). The subject of the discussion was Florentino, a sixty-seven-year-old retired Portuguese restaurant manager who had been ventilated with Covid for six weeks. He was still very sick. His lungs were stiff, his heart function was impaired, and his kidneys were completely reliant on artificial support. For weeks he seemed to have made no progress, and Mike wanted to check that we were doing the right thing. Should we really be continuing with full organ support for this patient?

A week previously I might have advocated continuing, purely to postpone another death, while not really believing that we would ever make him better, but now I was genuinely hopeful. I'd seen people in a worse state than Florentino pull through – not anyone who'd been so bad for so long perhaps, but still I believed he had a chance. I agreed that the odds were against him, but it was far from a done deal. As ever I was probably a bit over-excited and impassioned (verbose, even), but my colleagues didn't disagree. We should definitely carry on with full active, aggressive treatment. If things were getting worse in a week we could always reconsider.

I left the hospital that night with renewed energy and enthusiasm. Patients were getting better, it was VE Day, and the sun was shining in North London.

At home I discovered that Tish had arranged to have a socially distanced drink in the access path behind our house at the same time as our neighbours. I was immediately tetchy. I was sceptical that people would social distance, especially after a couple of glasses of Prosecco, and anyway I had spoken to plenty of people that day already. I was looking forward to catching up with the kids, a quick run and then the four of us eating together in the garden, but Tish had been living a very different life to me. She'd been cooped up at home for six weeks with two kids who were climbing the walls and she was desperate for some adult conversation (with someone other than me).

It turned out that the people she had arranged to 'near meet' were adults and so capable of resisting the urge to hug and slobber all over each other and they managed to stay at the ends of their own gardens. It was great. While the kids hung from trees and peppered us in Nerf gun pellets, we caught up with people we'd not really spoken to for months. We talked about the hospital briefly and inevitably they asked what I thought was going to happen next with Covid, but once we'd established that I had no more idea than they did, we moved on to other things. They too were struggling with home schooling and wrestling with how to persuade their parents to stick to the lockdown rules. We reflected on how lucky we were to have outside space and not have teenagers. We pondered the future – where we might go when we were allowed to travel again and how long the country would take to recover from the combined hits of Covid and Brexit – and then we all gently wandered back into our respective houses for some food.

At nine o'clock that evening an internationally renowned opera singer who lives at the other end of our street (this *is* North London) sang Vera Lynn songs from his balcony. I know almost nothing about opera (despite the fact that my brother directs it) and I had never heard Ian Bostridge sing before, but I stood in front of his house that night captivated. He wasn't singing loudly, but his voice floated over the warm evening air effortlessly, and I found it incredibly moving. It wasn't the song, pleasant as '(There'll Be Bluebirds Over) The White Cliffs Of Dover' is, or even what it represented, it was hearing somebody sing so beautifully, live, to Tish, me and a passing dog walker. I could have listened to him for hours. A few other couples paused on the street, and the neighbouring balconies filled, but unfortunately after three more songs he returned to his glass of wine and passed the baton to a group of talented amateurs from the house next door. After one final Nerf pellet each to the back of the neck, Tish and I decided to call it a night and headed for home. I wondered when we'd next hear live music.

The next day Boris announced that the message had changed.

We were in a new phase of the pandemic now, and rather than stay at home, save lives and protect the NHS we were to stay alert, control the virus and save lives. Some people, construction workers particularly, were actively encouraged to return to work if at all possible while others, if they could work at home, should do so; and everyone should bicycle – if they could – or drive, but definitely not take public transport – unless they needed to. I realized as I listened to the prime minister that, while I was not a particular fan of this government, I had been doing what I was told. Something in me still believed in their authority, and although I knew intellectually that what they'd been saying was a compromise and only one set of opinions, I wanted to believe it. I wanted to be told that it was OK to do this but not that and to have faith that someone knew what they were talking about. I'd been secretly hoping deep down that someone at the heart of government had a master plan and could see a clear way through this crisis. But with 'stay alert and control the virus' we seemed to be back in 'Brexit means Brexit' territory.

I was on a day off when we vacated the Pods on 10 May, but Elaine was there. She oversaw the repatriation of the final patients and staff from this pop-up ICU to the relative security of the permanent unit and then returned to the Pods, to help clear up. She moved furniture, cleaned equipment, returned items to their rightful places and then bid the whole place farewell. With the patients, staff and equipment gone, the Pods no longer existed, and in their place once again stood the operating theatres and recovery. For Elaine and many others, they had been a massive part of the pandemic, possibly the most dramatic, impressive and stressful element of the whole UCH response. She wanted to be there and see them safely shut down. She needed closure.

By the time I did my final night shift on 14 May, the ICU was unrecognizable. From a peak of over eighty-five ICU patients we were back down to twenty-eight. Many of the patients were still very sick, but this was like a normal night on ICU, except that in addition to the usual trainees, two consultant anaesthetists and I were on the night shift (we had waved goodbye to our GOSH colleagues four days previously). After handover the three of us had a cup of tea, caught up with each other's 'pandemics' and then embarked on a very civilized ward round. Trainees joined us and then fell away as we passed through their sections of the unit and I grumbled about some of the ventilatory strategies, but overall we changed very little. Jonathan, Florentino, Juan and Eli were all still sedated and ventilated but they were stable, and by 2 a.m. we had seen everyone. I even suggested that one of the anaesthetic consultants go home, but for logistical reasons neither could, so we had another cup of tea and then slunk off to various corners of the hospital to get some sleep. As I lay on my camp bed, under the desk, munching through a couple more of the seemingly endless supply of digestive biscuits and listening to the blinds flap noisily against the open window, I thought about how much things had changed in two weeks. The numbers were falling almost as quickly as they'd risen, and we couldn't stand staff down quickly enough. I thought back to Rik's debrief meeting and wondered what we'd actually do differently next time, what we'd really learned. We understood that it was a tricky, severe, unpredictable disease affecting not just the lungs, but the heart, kidneys and brain too. We knew that lots of the patients developed blood clots both big and small, some were very difficult to ventilate, some became hyper-inflamed, and some stayed sick for many weeks. We knew that we needed high-quality equipment and plenty of trained nurses to look after ICU Covid patients effectively, but we still didn't know which specific treatment strategies worked best. We knew that many patients, if they could ride out the worst, recovered in remarkable ways, but we also knew that many didn't make it. We'd lost more patients in the previous six weeks than at any other time in our careers.

Eventually I shut the window, moved the irritatingly loud ticking clock out into the hallway one last time and drifted into a fitful sleep.

Patients continued to make remarkable recoveries. Driton, our Brompton ECMO patient, was out of the unit two and a half weeks later, and Andrew recovered so quickly that he didn't even need a tracheostomy, despite being ventilated for over a month. That is almost unheard of in ICU. Juan, the nurse I'd turned on to his front, whilst cursing his tracheostomy, also suddenly turned the corner and escaped ICU in the first week of June.

Eli had played on my mind for days after his tracheostomy change and subsequent near cardiac arrest. I'd called his wife in and prepared her for the worst, but he held on for the next week and then gradually started to improve. Initially, when he was well enough to have his sedation lightened, he was delirious and, as with Thanasis, I worried that the forty minutes of low oxygen levels had damaged his brain, but in the end his confusion cleared as well, and on 1 June he was discharged to the ward. He was left with some weakness down his left side and after a month on the ward he was transferred to a specialist centre for neuro-rehabilitation. His wife sent us a lovely thank you card, which is pinned above the desk in our consultants' office. It still reminds me of that tracheostomy change and sends a shiver down my spine.

Fadi, the young man who'd been transferred to our sister hospital in Queen Square very early on, was home by mid-May, and Thanasis and Haydar were both discharged home in June.

Florentino, the subject of Alice, Mike and my three wise

people meeting, stayed on the ICU for seventy days. His lungs had seemed to .be stuck – stiff and irreversibly scarred – but through the second half of May something changed. We treated yet another chest infection and as usual set up a plan to try to wean him from the ventilator, and, rather than struggle for breath as he normally did, this time he responded. His kidneys sprang back into life, his lungs loosened up, and by 6 June he was free from all the machines and ready to be discharged to the ward. Less than two weeks later he was home.

Jonathan's battle with Covid continued throughout May. Some days he inched forward, and we were able to chip away at his support, but each time the improvement was followed by a seemingly inevitable setback. We continued to look for reversible problems and gave all the usual treatments, but we just couldn't get him well enough to breathe for himself. Throughout all this Megan remained at home shielding with the children, but the family liaison team set up regular video-link virtual visits.

Jonathan's body had been too weakened by the leukaemia and its treatments to fight Covid effectively, and in the third week of May his lungs deteriorated further. We looked for blood clots, we gave a course of antibiotics, we tried steroids, nitric oxide and various different modes of ventilation, but nothing made a significant difference. Within a few days his heart and then his kidneys began to fail too.

By 26 May Jonathan was on 100 per cent oxygen, high doses of heart stimulants and blood pressure support and 'the filter' for his kidneys. Najwan and Sam, the two ICU consultants looking after him through this period, were already considering whether ongoing treatment was futile, when one of Jonathan's pupils dilated and stopped constricting in response to light. Something significant had happened to Jonathan's brain, either a bleed or a clot.

That afternoon, despite the fact that his heart and lungs were still unstable on maximal support, Sam took Jonathan down for a CT scan of his head. The transfer was high risk, but they needed to know for sure, before talking to Megan. Unfortunately, the scan confirmed their worse fears. A clot was blocking a major blood vessel to Jonathan's brain, causing a catastrophic stroke. There was no way back for him now.

By chance the family liaison team on that day contained a neurologist, Richard, so he and Najwan set up a video call to break the news to Megan. Just as I had been all those weeks before, Najwan and Richard were deeply moved by the experience. Megan was in her bedroom this time. She had been through six weeks of torture and yet still she was composed and polite when she answered the call. She knew already that Jonathan was extremely unlikely to survive, but it was only now, with news of the stroke, that she realized all hope was gone, and tears began to roll down her cheeks. As she listened to Najwan and Richard, her children knocked innocently at her bedroom door to ask her questions. Najwan described it as heartrending to witness.

Richard set up one final bedside video call that evening, and Megan played videos to Jonathan from close family including the children. The last one was from her brother, a vicar, who administered the Last Rites.

A few minutes after the call Sam reduced the artificial organ support, and the focus of care shifted. The only priority now was to ensure that Jonathan was settled and comfortable. Shortly after eight o'clock on 26 May he died peacefully in his sleep with Richard and his ICU nurse, Taciana, holding his hand.

By the final week of May, it was clear that we were all but through the first surge. We were down to ten Covid ICU patients, and the unit was officially 'quiet', even by normal standards, but it turned out that recovering from a pandemic while simultaneously preparing for a possible second wave was a logistical nightmare. And so the meetings began.

These meetings weren't about a wave of patients flooding in through the front door tomorrow, though, they were about the details of how to return to normal in an uncertain and unpredictable future. They were filled with contingencies, risk stratification, financial constraints and public-private contracts. Local needs had to be played off against regional considerations, preparation for a second surge against business as normal, efficiency against safety. Rik found the meetings frustrating after his experience of the initial surge. A decision would be made and then a week later reversed, because it was impossible to make firm commitments on such shifting sands, so gradually he backed away from the larger organizational aspects and focused on specific projects such as an app he was building to monitor the hospital's daily oxygen consumption. Geoff and David (and others) pushed things forward, and services gradually started up again, but it was slow and laborious, and I was not envious of their days and weeks (months now) spent poring over complex and endlessly changing plans.

Alice, too, found this period tough. April had been a blur, during which she'd felt as if she was constantly rushing to keep up. If she wasn't clinical she was writing rotas or answering queries from trainees, but like the rest of us she was running on adrenaline. At the time her education bosses, Health Education England, were being very accommodating and hoped that the pandemic would not affect junior doctor training, but as Covid receded things started to change. Suddenly junior doctors' training *would* now be affected, and the reassurance she'd passed on to trainees was no longer valid. As well as fulfilling a full-time clinical commitment, she was fielding dozens of panicked phone calls a day, rewriting rotas, setting up a teaching programme in preparation for a second wave and worrying about her daughters, still 600 miles away on the Isle of Skye. As everyone else's lives calmed down, she seemed to be getting busier and began to feel frustrated and angry. Her daughters returned home on 20 May – not a minute too soon.

On 13 May, when 33,186 people had already died with Covid in the UK, Elaine attended a North London sector meeting with David to discuss what we'd all learned. It was supposed to be a chance for each hospital to share their experiences and insights, but Elaine says that she just sat there in silence. She felt empty and useless and was convinced that she had nothing to contribute. That night she sent a WhatsApp message to David: '. . . I've been struggling this week and just want to cry and having to hold back tears most of the time. Not really capable of having meaningful conversations . . . I'm so sorry for letting you down today.'

As David was quick to point out in his reply, she hadn't let anyone down. I am confident she spoke as much sense as anyone else at that meeting, but the previous two months had finally caught up with her. She had just led hundreds of nurses through the toughest experience of their careers and witnessed death and disease on a scale she'd never imagined. She'd not had a moment to process it all and finally it was catching up with her. Fortunately, Elaine has a wonderful husband and daughter at home whom she'd hardly seen for six weeks and some time off with them in Cambridgeshire gave her the breathing space she needed.

She says now that the pandemic has made her calmer and more pragmatic. When she goes to the big meetings to discuss budget cuts alongside expansion plans and the recruitment crisis, rather than feel frustrated, harassed and anxious, she takes it in her stride. She'll do what she can, and if that's not good enough, so be it. She shouldn't worry, it will always be more than good enough.

I wasn't suffering like Elaine and Alice, but I was starting to wonder what impact the pandemic had had on us. I wasn't really sure how I felt, let alone my colleagues. I had sat in Question and Answer sessions with the trainees, listened to the impact on my anaesthetic colleagues and was acutely aware of the enormous stress that all the nurses had been under, but what about us, the ICU consultants?

As a profession we are not very good at opening up about our mental health, but in the aftermath of Covid even we acknowledged that there might be issues to address. The difficulty was knowing how to go about it. There were drop-in sessions available and telephone numbers we could call, but we knew that none of us would, so eventually two colleagues (who had stayed away from Covid for health reasons) and a palliative care consultant approached the military. Trauma Risk Management (TRiM) is a peer-group-delivered procedure for soldiers who have been in stressful combat situations. It aims to keep staff functioning after traumatic experiences, educate and support those who need it and identify people requiring specialist support. My colleagues adapted TRiM for clinicians and renamed it Peer group REsilience Support System by dEbrief and Discussion (PRESSED – medics can't resist crow-barring in an acronym). They invited us to partake in groups of four. It was on Zoom and was scheduled to take between two and three hours.

In the end there were five ICU consultants on the call I joined, plus our two colleagues as facilitators. The structure was very straightforward. We each described ourselves before the pandemic (what we liked, what we did in our spare time, etc.), then how we felt during preparations, how that changed during the peak, and finally how we were getting on now in the aftermath. For the first time I really began to understand how different the experience had been for each of us, despite us all ostensibly doing the same job. Everyone opened up, and I learned things about my colleagues that I should have discovered years before, if only I'd taken the trouble to ask. It was interesting, moving and reassuring. And then Suzanne spoke.

Suzanne is Scottish but had trained in ICU and anaesthesia in Manchester. In early 2020, having finished her training, she'd decided to try a year of living it up in London before settling in the northwest, so in February she applied to join us as a locum consultant. We were impressed, offered her a job, and then Covid struck.

She hadn't started yet and she could easily have backed out and faced the crisis in a familiar hospital surrounded by her friends, but she didn't. She packed up her bags and her cat and set off for the epicentre of Covid, without even a flat to live in. She had made a commitment and she was going to stick to it. The hospital offered her temporary accommodation, and she started work, but to say it was tough is an understatement. She didn't know us, she didn't know how the hospital or the ICU worked, she didn't know the nurses, and any prospect of an induction was out of the window. She was in the middle of a pandemic in an alien environment and for her first three shifts she couldn't even log on to the computer. When she was off, even when she had found a flat, she could barely leave it.

As she told us all this on the Zoom call, tears began to stream down her face. For the previous two months she'd turned up to work with a smile and got on with it, so I had just assumed that she was coping. While many of us were huffing and puffing about how grim it all was, she seemed to be taking it in her stride. I may have offered the odd, 'You OK?' in passing but I'd never taken the time to sit down with her and really find out the answer. Superficially she was fine, and that was good enough for me.

Thankfully, as the rest of us mumbled sympathetic and apologetic words, her cat sashayed across her keyboard, flicked her face with its tail, and she laughed. Someone had got her back.

I left the session feeling that we should do something like this regularly, annually perhaps. It reminded me that setting time aside to talk to colleagues properly can be enormously powerful. Doctors are just not very good at doing it.

From February to June 2020 I didn't have a sniffle. I was as healthy as I have ever been. Obviously my hypochondria flared up intermittently, but there wasn't a single day on which even I could claim to be coming down with 'possible Covid'. I sat in a tightly packed office for weeks, rubbing shoulders with people who a day later tested positive. I spent two months in bays full of patients with it, and yet I had nothing.

One day in mid-May I was out running on the Heath, listening to Adam Buxton's weekly podcast, when he started talking to his guest about the possibility of a dystopian Covid society.

'We might split,' he mused, 'into the immune and the non-immune.'

The immune would carry medical ID and could travel freely and frequent pubs and restaurants, while the non-immune (the NI scum) would be restricted to their homes. PPE-clad police would roam the streets rounding up the scum and incarcerating them – for their own good. There would be a black market in fake 'immunity-ID' and secret underground gatherings of the NI resistance. There might be other groups, a shunned underclass of super spreaders, and ghostly shielders who'd not seen daylight for months. I have paraphrased and exaggerated (sorry Buckles), but the whole conversation unnerved me. It seemed far from certain that a vaccine would be developed, so we had to consider some form of long-term 'new normal'.

I concluded, along with Rik and Elaine, that I must have had Covid by now, but just been incredibly brave and not noticed (Alice had tested positive but suffered only mild symptoms). Rik was convinced that he'd had a slightly scratchy throat in

March, and Elaine had had one mild fever in early April, so we all waltzed in to have our antibody tests, confident of a positive result.

Jamie stabbed the end of my finger with a little too much enthusiasm and then squeezed three drops of blood on to the portable testing kit. I was completely relaxed as I waited for the two bands to appear across the white strip, one for the IgM antibody (indicating recent infection) and the other IgG (immunity).

'How's Vuppe?' I asked.

'You don't care.'

'I do, I feel sorry for her.'

Jamie looked up from the Covid test form he was filling out.

'What?' I asked innocently. 'She's obviously been terribly unwell.'

'Remind me how many times you took Tom and Edie to Casualty again, before they were one?'

'They are humans, to be fair.'

'Doggist.'

I glanced down at the white strip, but nothing had happened.

'Do you think it's deliberately like a pregnancy test?' I asked, starting to feel anxious but determined not to show it.

'Maybe you should try peeing on it.'

Five minutes later the strip was still white.

'How reliable is this kit? Is it just some cheap shit you picked up off the internet?'

'Umm,' Jamie was backing away from me now, trying not to laugh. 'No.' He paused. 'It can take ten minutes. Why don't you take it away with you?'

'How many have you done?'

'Forty.'

'And?'

'All the people who've had confirmed Covid have come up positive, but only two others.'

'Seriously?'

This couldn't be right. I must have had Covid, I'd been living in a soup of it for two months. I stormed back to our office and put the test strip on the desk next to my computer. Over the next half an hour I pretended to work while glancing furtively at the strip every three or four minutes. It remained determinedly white, so I decided not to believe Jamie's kit. It was odd, admittedly, that Rik, Elaine, David, Dave and Steve had also all turned up negative – that was a lot of false negatives, but maybe theirs were correct. All I knew was that mine couldn't be.

The next week I took a different test, the official one, bought by the hospital. This wasn't some cheap knock-off kit picked up by Jamie for a tenner, it was the most accurate test available. And I was negative again: nothing, not a whiff of either antibody.

I was gutted. After two months surrounded by Covid, I was still as vulnerable as when we'd started. It seemed so unfair. I'd still have to be as careful, still consider every patient a threat, still avoid crowded shops, public transport and my parents. I couldn't justify going to see them, knowing I might pick up the virus at any time. In six weeks I'd be fifty and move into a higher-risk group. I'd thought I was immune, invincible, but actually I was just gradually becoming more vulnerable.

Most of us had planned to have time off when it was over and head somewhere nice to put our feet up and be pampered. I was meant to be in France for the May half-term, chilling out at my sister's house and forgetting all about it, but the country was still in lockdown. We were allowed to take unlimited exercise outside and sunbathe, but hotels and pubs were not due to open until July, and non-essential international travel was still banned. Taking a holiday meant staying at home with the odd trip to a local park, so few people seized the opportunity. By chance we had a family holiday in Scotland booked at the end of July. It coincided well with the plans to ease the lockdown, so we decided to stick with that.

Eventually I put the disappointment of my antibody test behind me and started to relax. Alice and I had written a new rota for June and July, the sun was shining, and we'd done OK. It was time to stop worrying about the 'what ifs', accept my antibody status and move on.

I was at home when Elaine phoned me on 26 May.

'Hi, Elaine, how's it going? Good bank holiday?'

'Yes, thanks. You?'

'Yeah, fine. We did a day trip to Tish's parents' farm, but they couldn't let us into the house so . . . Anyway, what can I do for you?'

'I'm sorry to bother you at home.'

'Don't be silly. Are you OK?'

'Yeah, I am, but . . .' Elaine paused. 'There's been a cluster of Covid amongst the nursing staff.'

'Our nursing staff? I mean ICU nurses?'

'Yeah.'

'Oh God.' My heart sank. 'Are they OK?'

'Most of them are fine.'

'Most?'

'Tess is up on the ward on oxygen.'

'Right.'

'And Carla is not well. I think she's going to come in.'

We sat in silence for a moment as the news sank in. Tess was fifty-three years old and Carla thirty-five. Both were healthy, and both had been working on the UCH ICU for the previous three months.

'How many others have tested positive?'

'Seven, with another four possibles.'

'Do they live together?'

'No, they were all on a night shift two weeks ago.'

'I'm so sorry, Elaine. I'm on the unit tomorrow.'

'I know.'

'I'll go up and see Tess.'

'That would be great, thanks. I've been texting. She's OK, but she's on 50 per cent oxygen.'

'Do you need me to say something at the morning brief?'

'No, no . . . I'll do that.'

'Do you think this is the . . .' I couldn't face even saying the words. We hadn't admitted a new Covid patient to ICU for over a week.

'Let's hope not,' said Elaine. 'I'm going to start the contact tracing in the morning.'

When I saw Tess the next morning with her infectious diseases consultant, she was coping well. She was moderately breathless and had been on CPAP for short periods, but for most of the time she was stable on 50 per cent oxygen via a normal facemask. We offered her the option of transfer to ICU, but she was keen to avoid it if at all possible, so we agreed to keep her where she was with regular review from our team. By the following day, however, she was worse. She now needed continuous CPAP, and we all agreed it was time to bring her down into the ICU.

We offered Tess the option of transferring to a different hospital, to be cared for by people she didn't know, but she chose to stay with us. Although there are drawbacks to being looked after by your colleagues (natural reflexes risk being overriden by hyper-vigilance and over-thinking), I would have made the same decision.

We needed to consider the impact on all the other staff. The nurses and doctors were exhausted, physically and mentally, and we had no idea how they would cope with seeing one of their own so sick. What if, God forbid, she continued to deteriorate?

Anyone who felt uncomfortable was not asked to look after

Tess, but plenty of her colleagues volunteered. We limited access to her electronic records to maintain her confidentiality and reminded everyone to respect her dignity and privacy. No one needed reminding; all of us could imagine ourselves in her shoes.

For four days Tess sat clamped to her CPAP mask. Her oxygen requirement increased to 60 per cent, then dipped a bit, then increased again. Her blood markers of inflammation rose, but not catastrophically high, and we wrestled with all the usual dilemmas. Should we give her antibiotics? Should we give her steroids, or anti-virals? When would be the right time to consider intubation? In the end we gave antibiotics, because of her high inflammatory markers, but not steroids or anti-virals, because she'd already joined a clinical trial of a powerful anti-inflammatory, Ruxolitinib.

And then we watched and waited. It was up to the virus now, and her immune system. We knew by this stage that about half of patients who required CPAP went on to need intubation, and, once intubated, her chances of surviving were not much better than fifty-fifty.

Thankfully, after four long days on the unit, her breathing improved. Her oxygen requirements reduced, her inflammatory blood markers settled, and she started to tolerate time off the CPAP. Two days after that, she was completely free from it, twenty-four hours a day. Her lungs were recovering, and her heart and kidneys had come through unscathed.

But the following day we admitted Carla. She was now breathing hard and required CPAP, so we began the whole process again. Carla's blood markers were never as high as Tess's, so we held off antibiotics, but she received the anti-viral Remdesivir and also signed up to the trial of Ruxolitinib. Her breathing seemed more laboured than Tess's, and she spent many hours curled forward onto her front, trying to optimize the performance of her lungs. The anxiety with Carla was not so much her gas exchange, but the effort it took for her to breathe. For several days she looked and felt exhausted, but eventually, after a tense week of CPAP, she too turned the corner.

None of us know whether Carla or Tess received Ruxolitinib or a placebo. We don't know if Tess's antibiotics helped or Carla's anti-virals. Neither received steroids, the first group of drugs to show benefit in Covid, or plasma exchange, or any other trial drugs, but I suspect that none of those therapies, or lack of them, was crucial. I think Tess and Carla were just unlucky to get so sick from Covid in the first place and then lucky to receive excellent care and recover.

All of the other ICU nurses who caught Covid recovered without coming into hospital, and the outbreak spread no further. This turned out to be just a cluster, but it was also a timely reminder. This was not over. An outbreak like ours could happen again at any time. We were still living with Covid and would be for the foreseeable future.

Even before the first wave was over, a second wave was in the back of our minds. Whilst desperate to believe that it might not materialize or that by some miracle a vaccine might be produced by the autumn, we knew that in all likelihood Covid was coming back. Mixed in with other winter viruses, the overall impact of another wave could be worse than the first. For a time in the first surge everyone focused on Covid, but the second time around the pressure to maintain normal, non-Covid treatments would be greater because the backlog of patients was already there. Running Covid and non-Covid side by side would be complex and hazardous.

We would be better prepared for the disease, though. We might have little clinical trial evidence, but we'd have our experience and the experience of hundreds of other hospitals around the country and the world. By the next surge we'd have local and national clinical guidelines, we'd have more ICU ventilators, more CPAP beds and more staff with ICU experience to call on. We would know what to expect.

Rik discharged our final Covid patient (of the first surge) out of ICU on 27 June. That afternoon he took the white sheets off the walls. We no longer needed our Covid ICU floor plan, with its orange and purple Vs and Cs; we hadn't had a proper SitRep meeting for weeks. Just as Elaine had felt compelled to close down the Pods in person, so Rik needed to convert the SitRep command centre back into the ICU seminar room.

When we finally analysed the data, it emerged that our patients did roughly as well as those in most other large centres. Approximately two-thirds of our critically sick Covid patients survived. Like everyone, we got better at treating the disease as the pandemic progressed. We learned as we gained experience, and our outcomes improved, but I was pleased to see that our efforts were consistent throughout. We pushed as hard and for as long with patients at the beginning of the pandemic as we did during the peak and after it.

Comparisons between hospitals are always difficult because, like schools, what you get out depends to an extent on what you put in. If we admitted lots more older and sicker patients than another hospital, then we'd expect our mortality to be higher. Statisticians could correct for that to a degree, but with Covid the picture was more complicated. Some hospitals were hit by a tsunami of patients very early on and ran out of capacity and resources within a few days. Others had a later, slower influx so they had more time to learn and prepare. In addition, patients moved between hospitals. Often the more stable patients were transferred from the smaller hospitals to the bigger ones, leaving behind the sicker patients who were less likely to survive. Added to that, resource was not spread evenly between sites. Some hospitals could mobilize research staff, some (like us) were offered help by neighbouring trusts, some had a huge estate, lots of equipment and plenty of oxygen, but many had none of these things. This was not a level playing field. Certain hospitals may have got more right and done some things better, but there were myriad explanations for the variability in outcomes. We should all try to learn, but hospitals that did well should be wary of self-congratulation, and those that didn't should not beat themselves up too much. We all faced a unique set of challenges in very different circumstances.

I made it down to Dorset to see my parents at the end of June. I was nervous about the train journey, particularly about picking up the virus on the way down and passing it on to Mum and Dad, so I wore a full FFP3 mask and wiped the surfaces at least every hour, but the train was empty. I had the carriage almost to myself and apart from changing on to the wrong train at Bournemouth and heading briefly back towards London, the journey was extremely pleasant.

Mum's dementia had inevitably progressed, but her face lit up when I walked in through the front door. We played tennis, and although initially she tried to hit the ball tin rather than the ball itself, once settled, we played solidly for over an hour. The harder I hit the ball, the harder it came back. It was a joy to see her mind clear as years of muscle memory took over, and we both walked off the court exhausted but smiling.

When I was a child, my Dad used to talk about people who'd had 'a good war'. I didn't understand; it seemed a perverse concept to me, a contradiction in terms. Surely there was no such thing as 'a good war'. War was awful – for everyone. But through the spring and summer, as the pandemic progressed, the military metaphors used to discuss it stacked up – battles were won and lost, there were heroes and victims, survivors and casualties. I started to think about the phrase and consider whether I, and the ICU, could venture to say we had had a 'good pandemic'. I thought we could. We had been frightened and anxious, deeply upset at times, but that first surge was without doubt the biggest challenge of our careers, and the sense of purpose and achievement was undeniable. We'd been at the heart of it from the start, facing an unprecedented threat, and we'd come through it. Not unscathed – I had got things wrong, was haunted by some of the decisions I had made, and the prospect of another winter surge filled me with dread – but we had shared a cataclysmic experience, we'd been pushed to our limits and we'd not been overwhelmed by it. The support and camaraderie on those night shifts was like nothing I'd previously experienced in medicine. I saw the best of my co-workers and, at times, of myself. I was beginning to understand what my dad meant.

Epilogue

In September 2020 I telephoned the families of the deceased to ask permission to include their loved ones in this book. It turned out to be an educational and humbling experience.

Adam's mother was generous and accommodating, despite having suffered painful press intrusion following Adam's death. She described Adam as a 'great son and devoted father, who was missed desperately by the whole family'. She also told me that she had been overwhelmed by the number of people who had contacted her after his death to tell her how kind and generous Adam had been to them. He was, she said, 'a people person and a gentleman, who had made her so proud'.

Tricia's husband Andy described both Tricia and the process of losing the love of his life with heartbreaking insight and candour. He said that Tricia adored her job at GOSH. She was a force of nature, combining a natural ease around children with an intellect and determination that led to publication in *The Lancet*. She embodied the GOSH motto – 'The child first and always' – but also brought just as much fearless vigour and energy to her other roles of school governor and magistrate. She was also a wonderful mother, and life had been unbearably hard at times since her death, but despite that Andy was grateful to have had the chance to spend so much time with his two precious children over the subsequent six months.

At the end of the call he told me a quick story. Last year, Luke, their son, had applied to join the navy but failed the eyesight test due to an abnormality of his colour perception and so was rejected. Tricia, who'd taken him for the test, was not at all convinced by the process and left determined to take him back for a second go. Tragically, Covid intervened, but as so often, she was right. Luke passed his repeat eyesight test in the summer of 2020 with flying colours and is off next year to fulfil his dream.

Andy, Emily and Luke added these words: 'The passage of time since our cruel loss of Tricia does not assuage the pain each one of us feels but we will honour her memory by letting the wisdoms she left with us in life guide us towards a better future.'

Megan wrote the following about Jonathan:

Jonathan was very well travelled, he spent a lot of time touring with his work as a lighting designer, director and programmer, a job he loved and was hugely admired for in the industry.

His artistic eye and musicality, along with his attention to detail and precision provided many rock'n'roll and huge live events with amazing lighting in stadiums all over the world.

Despite his demanding job and no matter where he was in the world, he always had time for his family and he was happiest at home.

His dedication and love for me and our lovely children was enormous and he was so proud of us all. I honestly couldn't have wished for a more amazing husband or a more loving father to our children. He would do anything for us all with masses of love, generosity and determination.

He was incredibly strong and over the course of his illness he amazed me with his determination, positivity and ability to be calm under pressure, all this along with a total lack of complaining throughout the toughest of challenges.

He fought so very hard.

Myself and the children will continue to do him proud.

I'd like to take this opportunity to say an enormous thank you to all of the NHS staff at UCLH, who showed, along with all their knowledge and expertise, such amazing kindness and care to Jonathan throughout his treatments. This extended to me and once Jonathan was on the ventilator they provided me with a chance to support and comfort him from afar which was incredibly important. All of this was enormously appreciated and won't be forgotten.

I would like to thank them again for their patience and generosity and for allowing me to tell a small fragment of their loved ones' stories.

Then I moved on to the survivors. They were amazing. They'd suffered horribly, and some were still struggling, but to a person they were determined to be positive. They were not going to be defined by Covid.

John, the easygoing publican who'd narrowly avoided the ventilator, was back working forty to fifty hours a week in the Green Man. He was still breathless when he exerted himself, but otherwise his life was back to normal, and he was particularly grateful for the return of live sport.

Thanasis, who shouted 'HELLO LONDON!' to the BBC, travelled back to his home town of Larissa in Greece for six weeks over the summer to witness the birth of his first grandchild. I spoke to his wife, Eleni, on their return. She described him as positive and grateful, but he still had problems. He used to love walking but could only make it round his local park now with a frame and was not able to return to work because he had foot drop, which prevented him from driving. He did his best not to show it, she said, because he was a strong, proud man who did not want his family to feel sad or sorry for him, but he found life after Covid hard. He was, however, determined and optimistic about the future.

Fadi, the young man whom we had transferred to our sister hospital, proved to me that he was back running his café/restaurant while we were on the phone by asking me to hold the line while he served a customer. Times were hard, though, and his staff had gone down from four pre-Covid to one. He still got breathless climbing stairs and was troubled by unpleasant and confusing flashbacks, but generally he was improving, feeling positive and determined to get on with it – he had a business to run and a daughter to support.

Haydar, the man Mervyn, Rik and I had the three wise people discussion about, was improving all the time, his daughter told me, and delighted to be able to walk down his street again unaided. His family tied a thank you letter to the post outside the front entrance of UCH. It was there for weeks and lifted the spirits of countless staff members. He was planning a holiday for 2021 but for now was happy just to be at home surrounded by his loving and protective family.

Syrie, the non-Covid patient whose dad I know, has avoided hospital ever since. Life has continued to be tough, because she has had to be careful and stay in a lot, but she did get away to Scotland in the summer with her family. She is now preparing for her Mandarin and Biology A levels. (English is already in the bag) with the goal of studying Korean at the School of Oriental and African Studies at London University. She'd planned to visit South Korea on the anniversary of her liver transplant, but will now go in 2021 instead. She said that one thing the pandemic had done was give people an insight into an aspect of life with chronic illness. Suddenly people couldn't do what they wanted, their options were limited. For much of the time they were stuck at home, like many people with chronic illness are throughout their lives.

Juan, the elderly care nurse with the early tracheostomy, whom I'd turned in the middle of the night, was back home with his wife and eight-year-old grandson. He refused to admit that he had any sequelae of Covid and had recently started jogging again in

Regent's Park. He was still awaiting clearance to return to work but was confident it would come through soon. He felt ready.

Eli (the trachey change) spent a total of twenty-two weeks in hospital. His recovery was complicated by significant weakness of his left arm and leg, but when I spoke to him in September 2020 he was walking around the house unaided and outside for half an hour with a stick. He described himself as 'the Miracle Boy', and I couldn't disagree. He said that he still struggled to find the occasional word, but he sounded sharp on the phone. He wasn't back to work at his development construction company yet but he was just starting to involve himself again with children's charity Zichron Menachem.

When Andrew, the young IT manager who'd self-proned for days on his plasma exchange, answered the phone it was hard to believe he had ever been so ill, or even ill at all. His voice was crisp, he was back at work almost full-time and he planned to have his Sorrento wedding celebration in June 2021. He'd suffered with painful ankles that had limited his exercise, but they were improving every day. Prior to Covid he'd been a passionate offshore yacht racer and towards the end of summer 2020 he'd managed to get out sailing again – not offshore racing yet, but it was a big step in the right direction.

Driton, the Kosovan plasterer with air around his heart who'd gone for ECMO, was back home living with his wife and two children by the time I called. He had been breathless when first discharged from hospital, but by the summer he was able to go hill-walking in his native Kosovo. He still suffered with muscle pains after exercise but was now able to run two miles and had recently returned to work as a plasterer.

Florentino's son Pedro had just reopened 'Otino's', his father's old restaurant in Camden when I called. Florentino (the man Alice, Mike and I discussed, who was on the ICU for seventy days) was still limited to his home and balcony, but he was delighted to be spending time with his five young grandchildren and he too had a big trip planned for 2021. He wanted to feel the sand between his toes on the beaches near his hometown of Sintra in Portugal.

Finally, to Tess and Carla, our two ICU nurses. I can't imagine what was going through their minds when they were moved down to the ICU, having looked after Covid patients for two months. When I called in August, however, both were doing well. Carla had continued to be breathless for weeks and had felt very low at times, and Tess was still short of breath when she exercised, had pain under her rib cage and suffered with low mood and guilt, but every day things were improving. They spoke openly and candidly to me, and although they were still finding it tough, I was left feeling optimistic. They are both admirable and inspirational nurses. Carla was already on a phased return to work, and Tess planned to follow her two weeks later; both heading back to their jobs in the UCH ICU.

Afterword

We are in a lull. It is late May 2021 as I write this, and only three of the 295 Covid patients we admitted to ICU during the recent surge remain on the unit, all now testing negative. We have not admitted a new case for over a month. I am hoping that this will turn into more than a lull and become the new normal, but already there are cases in ICUs in the northwest of England, and the modellers are predicting a third wave as soon as July.

The second surge was very much like the first one, with some differences. We transferred 141 ventilated Covid patients into our ICU from other hospitals, transformed theatres into another pop-up ICU, converted a medical ward into a further twenty ICU beds and two other wards into CPAP units. We had a clearer idea of what to expect, so we were better organized, but the speed and scale of the second wave was shocking. The new variant spread much more quickly than anyone had predicted.

In some ways the work was less onerous. Once again, ICU was the centre of attention, and staff from all over the hospital flooded back through our doors to help. Consultant surgeons and medical students took regular shifts as ICU nursing assistants, dentists ran our family liaison team, and crack proning teams roamed the units. We had the equipment, oxygen, electricity and emergency rotas ready to go, there were now a couple of drugs that had been shown to improve Covid outcomes, and we knew and trusted the PPE. We went back on to night shifts, but this time there were two ICU consultants present overnight, so the stress and responsibility were shared.

The problem was that my expectations were too high. Having seen such remarkable recoveries towards the end of the first wave, I thought that if we were just determined and persistent then this time round we'd be able to save more people. Patients came back from the brink first time round, from past the brink, from places I'd thought were beyond hope. Never give up, I reasoned, and eventually they'd pull through – not all of them perhaps, but the vast majority. I was wrong. The outcomes were better than in the first surge, but not dramatically so. More people caught Covid this time, so more came to ICU and more died. They didn't die in the first surge because we gave up on them, they died because Covid is brutal and relentless, and while some patients claw their way back against the odds, many do not – whatever support and care they receive. Second time round, I found this harder to accept. Like many of the relatives, I couldn't let go. Even when there was no longer any realistic hope, I wanted to persist and drive the organs on rather than accept reality and switch the focus to delivering comfort and dignity.

There were remarkable and uplifting stories. A woman in her thirties with several chronic health problems who was on maximal multiple organ support for weeks, and on three occasions came within a whisker of dying, left the unit with everything in working order and a huge smile on her face; the mother of one of the nurses, ventilated for five weeks, is now home and well on the way to a full recovery; and a man in his forties, on the ICU for over three months, has just achieved his first twenty-four hours free from the ventilator. There are many more stories of survival against the odds, but another group has also stayed with me – the people who did not want to be ventilated.

By the new year of 2021, many people knew that if you ended up on a ventilator with Covid you could very well die. As a result some patients were determined to avoid it. They'd rather sit panting on CPAP masks for days than go off to sleep – however hard we tried to persuade them otherwise. We still didn't know the optimal time to change over, but now we were grappling with the added complication of people refusing to follow our advice anyway – until they were so ill that they lost consciousness.

'At that point,' they said, 'you can put me on the ventilator.' We tried to explain that we thought this would increase the risks, but we had no evidence to prove it, and it was their bodies not ours, so in the end it was their decision. Our job was to advise and offer treatments, not to force those treatments on people against their will. This was troubling and frustrating, but I was sympathetic to their position. I have little sympathy for anti-vaxxers and anti-maskers who put their own and other people's lives at risk on the basis of misinformation and conspiracy theories, but this group was different. While awake, these patients still had a semblance of control. They were actively participating in the struggle to get better, but once asleep and on a ventilator they ceded all power and responsibility to us. Normally patients have had enough by the time we suggest ventilating them, but with Covid's 'happy hypoxia' some patients still felt reasonably well despite looking awful and having frighteningly low oxygen levels.

I am still in touch with several of the patients and families that I wrote about in *Life Support*. Megan requested a copy of the book and then texted to say: 'I am proud that Jonathan and I are a small part of your book. It is written with much care and thought for all involved and clearly comes from the heart.' It was the only review I needed, and I replied to thank her and added that I would love to go and see her next theatrical production. 'That would be great,' she replied. So it's a date (just not a specific one yet).

I was walking to my car after a thirteen-hour day shift in February when Tricia's daughter Emily called me. She wanted to discuss the topic that she'd been asked to prepare for her medical school interview. She thought I might have some insights.

'Sure,' I agreed. 'What's the subject?'

'The medical ethics of a pandemic.'

'Wow . . . Gosh!' I answered, eloquently. 'Tough. How are you all?'

'We're OK,' she replied, as calm and composed as ever. For the next half an hour I sat in the front seat of my car discussing the medical ethics of the Covid pandemic with the bereaved daughter of one of its victims. I don't think I told her much that she didn't already know, but I am delighted (and relieved) to confirm that she will be starting medical school in the autumn. I had to fight back tears when she told me that her long-term goal was to become a paediatrician. Perhaps one day she'll work in her mother's hospital.

I joined a webinar with Eli (the man with the tracheostomy and the near fatal pneumothorax) in February. People from around the world had tuned in to hear him tell his remarkable Covid story, and at his request I had recorded a short video describing the fateful day of his pneumothorax and my subsequent conversation with his wife. Having endured my own awkward performance, I sat back to listen to Eli and found myself transfixed by the bright, animated face on the screen. It was so many miles from the pale, lifeless one that had been stuck in that ICU bed for all those weeks. We are still in touch, and he continues to improve. His eyes and hands still bother him, but he has discovered gyms and burpees for the first time in his life, and his determination knows no bounds. He really is 'the miracle boy'.

Tess was back working in the non-Covid ICU during the second surge, but Carla returned to the Covid ICU. Occasionally I wondered what she must be thinking as she looked after yet another Covid patient who was clinging to life, but she seemed to be just getting on with it.

On 29 January, Elaine, the ICU matron, sent an email to ICU staff. We were at the height of the second wave, with almost 120 Covid patients in the various ICUs, and many of the staff were at breaking point. The email's attachment was a thank you letter from Andrew, the recently married IT manager and offshore yacht sailor from surge one. His timing could not have been better. As well as thanking us all profusely, he informed us that he was back to working full-time and living a pretty normal life (as far as lockdown permitted). He included pictures of him and his wife arm in arm on a winter walk along the Thames. He explained how he now appreciated the smaller things in life, like sunlight through a window and his nephew's pride in the cave he had built with a blanket across the sofa for a Zoom call. At the end of his letter Andrew told us a secret; his wife was twenty-one weeks' pregnant with their first child.

I have still not had Covid and I have now had both doses of the vaccine. None of my close family have had Covid either, but at the end of March 2021 we admitted my mother to a nursing home. Her dementia had progressed to the point where my father and the home carers could no longer look after her safely. She was still physically fit, able to walk miles through the Dorset hills, which made dropping her off even more heartbreaking. We tried to explain the situation to her, but she didn't understand, and although I speak to her regularly on the telephone, I think she only recognizes my voice fleetingly. Often she becomes agitated or tearful during the calls. I'm not allowed to visit because of Covid, but my father is permitted to go in once every ten days for an hour, and now my brother can join him. I feel helpless, angry, guilty and desperately sad, but I'm aware that there are millions like me. It's just another legacy of this horrible virus.

In February 2021, I was interviewed by Andrew Billen of *The Times*. At the end of the piece he postulated that he had met a sadder and wiser Jim Down than he would have a year previously. My sister firmly disagreed on both counts, but it made me wonder whether the past year has changed me. My daughter thinks I have lost some joy and silliness. She said to me in March 2021 that I am less likely to laugh, less likely to say funny things and less patient with her and her brother's tomfoolery.

I think that she is right. I have always been anxious and impatient, but previously these tendencies were offset by my ability to switch off for periods and to allow my puerile sense of humour and half-baked opinions free rein. I loved sitting in the garden with a beer, chatting and laughing with family and friends. I could do it for hours – putting the world to rights, exchanging insults and talking nonsense – but in the past year I'd properly relaxed and let go perhaps three or four times. I'd almost always been preoccupied with work or my parents or catching Covid or spreading Covid or whether we were failing at home schooling or writing *Life Support*. I'd stopped messing about, and it was time to start again. I was infuriated to have to admit that my eleven- (albeit going on sixteen-) year-old daughter had so easily seen what I'd been oblivious to, so please don't tell her (there is little danger that she'll read this).

It seems, therefore, that Covid has made me sadder – temporarily I hope. But has it made me wiser? I think one thing it has taught me is to accept what I don't know. Dealing with a brand-new disease, particularly one so prevalent and severe, forced us to embark on treatment strategies that we knew might be wrong. There was no hedging of bets. We had to do something and we'd only find out much later (if ever) whether we had picked the right options. We made speculative decisions on an unprecedented scale during Covid, but the truth is that ICU doctors make decisions every day without 'knowing' the right answer. All doctors do. We might know the best option for a population with a certain condition, or the prognosis for a group of similar people with the same diagnosis, but we rarely know categorically what is best for the particular patient in front of us. Sometimes we are 99 per cent sure, and the decision is straightforward, but often we are using an imperfect mix of evidence, guidelines, experience and intuition to formulate a plan. We suggest treatments that we think are in the patient's best interests, but it is important to remember that, however expert we are, in the end often we are only offering our opinion. Covid has reminded me of that.

The UK has fewer ICU beds per head of population than the USA and most equivalent European countries. Every winter we are pushed to the limit and we postpone hundreds of major operations due to lack of ICU capacity. In London we struggle to staff the beds we have, and Brexit has only made things worse. One positive legacy of the pandemic may be that we create more beds and recruit more nurses. We need flexibility to deal with a future pandemic, but we also need an adequate bed base to cope with normal winter pressures. The pandemic has taken its toll on the nurses (in the event of another surge this autumn our workforce might be our most vulnerable resource) but it has also reminded the public what a vital and extraordinary job they do. From the recent recruitment figures it would seem that people want to become nurses again.

But resources will always be finite. In some ways ICU has been relatively protected up to now. If I want to admit and ventilate someone (or, if we are full, transfer them out to an ICU that has a bed), no one will stop me. No one will question my use of £1,700 per day of taxpayers' money. I try to admit patients who I think have a reasonable chance of recovering to a meaningful quality of life, but no one has defined reasonable chance or meaningful quality of life. Each ICU doctor has a different perspective, depending on his or her background, experience, personality and biases. They are further influenced by their emotions on the day, the threat of future criticism, the strength of opinion from the family and the competition for beds. As technology advances and new treatments are developed, these decisions will only become more pressing and difficult.

Post-Brexit and post-pandemic, we have to ask ourselves what the future of healthcare in Britain might look like. Where does the ICU fit into this vision? What do we want it to do and where is it on the priority list? How do we ensure that, when the next crisis comes, we are ready?

Glossary

Blood gas

A bedside blood test that measures the levels of oxygen, carbon dioxide, acid, haemoglobin, sodium and potassium in the blood.

'Bloods'

Colloquial term for blood tests, used to measure blood cell counts, electrolytes and other molecules in the blood.

COVID-19 (Covid)

COronaVIrus Disease 2019. Disease caused by SARS-CoV 2 and discovered in 2019.

CPAP

Continuous Positive Airway Pressure. Constant positive pressure applied via a mask or hood to the mouth and nose.

CRP

C Reactive Protein. A blood marker of inflammation typically very high in severe Covid.

CT scanner

Medical scanner that gives cross-sectional images of parts or all of the body. Sometimes referred to as a 'CAT' scanner.

The Doppler	A probe that passes through the mouth into the oesophagus to measure blood flow out of the heart.
EAU	Emergency Assessment Unit.
ECG	Electrocardiogram. A recording of the electrical activity of the heart via sensors on the skin. ECGs detect the rhythm and rate of the heartbeat and identify abnormalities such as heart attacks.
Echocardiogram	Ultrasound scan to look at the structure and function of the heart.
ECMO	ExtraCorporeal Membrane Oxygenation. A machine to oxygenate blood and remove carbon dioxide in a circuit outside of the body.
ED	Emergency Department (also known as A and E and Casualty).
Encephalitis	Inflammation of the brain sometimes caused by viruses.
ENT	Ear Nose and Throat.
Endotracheal tube	A breathing tube that passes through the mouth down into the windpipe (trachea).
FFP3 mask	Filtering Face Pieces 3 mask. A mask that protects against viruses, bacteria and fungal spores.

The 'filter'	ICU 'dialysis type' machine that takes over the function of the kidneys when they cease to function adequately.
GIK	Glucose, insulin and potassium. A combination of infusions to improve the heart function.
GOSH	Great Ormond Street Hospital.
Haematologist	Doctor specializing in blood. Some sub-specialize in blood cancer, others in blood clotting, others in sickle cell disease, etc.
HASU	Hyper-Acute Stroke Unit.
HDRU	High-Dependency Respiratory Unit.
ICU	Intensive Care Unit (also known as Intensive Therapy Unit (ITU) and Critical Care Unit (CCU).
Lymphocyte	A type of white blood cell, typically low in Covid patients.
Meningitis	Infection of the lining of the brain.
Microbiologist	Doctor who specializes in the bacteria and other micro-organisms that cause infections.
Peri-operative medicine	The medical care of patients before, during and after high-risk surgery.
The Pods	A makeshift ICU in the operating theatre complex.

PPE	Personal protective equipment.
Registrar	Middle-grade doctor between SHO and consultant.
Resus	Resucitation room in the Emergency Department.
SARS-CoV 2	Severe Acute Respiratory Syndrome Coronavirus 2, so called because the virus is related to the coronavirus that caused SARS in 2003.
SHO	Senior house officer, junior training doctor.
SOP	Standard Operating Procedure.
Tracheostomy	Breathing tube placed through the front of the neck into the windpipe.
UCH	University College Hospital, part of University College London Hospitals NHS Trust.

Acknowledgements

Thank you first to all the patients and relatives of patients for allowing me to include you in this book. Your strength and courage is extraordinary, and you have taught me so much. Thanks also to my wonderful colleagues at UCH, particularly in ICU, theatres and anaesthetics. I am lucky to work in such a friendly and inspiring hospital.

Thank you to George Collee, Tiffany Murray, Belinda Jones, Sharon Hughff, Elliot Levey, Harry Mackrill, John Burgess, Tom Connolly, Edward Docx and James Wood for teaching me to write and encouraging me along the way.

I am indebted to Georgia Garrett for her faith, wisdom and guidance and also to Katie Haines and Honor Spreckley. Thank you to my brilliant editors Venetia Butterfield and Tom Killingbeck for so carefully and cleverly knocking this book into shape and to Isabel Wall, Amelia Fairney, Poppy North and Olivia Mead at Viking for your help and support.

Thank you to Rosie Blau, Rik Thomas, Alice Carter, Monty and Kate Mythen, Elaine Thorpe, Ramani Moonesinghe, Irene Bouras, David Howell, Sam Clarke, Dave Brealey, Sharon Spitteri, Viki Mitchell, Steve Harris and James Holding for reading and editing early drafts. Oh, and thanks to Jamie Smart, I suppose.

Thank you to my wonderful family, Peter Down, Maddy Down, Mark Down and Caroline Filippin. Finally, eternal thanks to Edie, Tom and my wife Tish for your love and patience. You are the world to me.